Improving Palliative Care for Cancer
Summary and Recommendations

Kathleen M. Foley and Hellen Gelband, *Editors*

National Cancer Policy Board

INSTITUTE OF MEDICINE

and

NATIONAL RESEARCH COUNCIL

NATIONAL ACADEMY PRESS
Washington, D.C.

NATIONAL ACADEMY PRESS • 2101 Constitution Avenue, N.W. • Washington, DC 20418

NOTICE: The project that is the subject of this report was approved by the Governing Board of the National Research Council, whose members are drawn from the councils of the National Academy of Sciences, the National Academy of Engineering, and the Institute of Medicine. The members of the Board responsible for the report were chosen for their special competences and with regard for appropriate balance.

Support for this project was provided by the National Cancer Institute; the Centers for Disease Control and Prevention; the American Cancer Society; American Society of Clinical Oncology; Abbott Laboratories; Amgen, Inc.; and Aventis. The views presented in this report are those of the Institute of Medicine and Commission on Life Sciences National Cancer Policy Board and are not necessarily those of the funding agencies.

International Standard Book Number 0-309-07563-7

Additional copies of this report are available for sale from the National Academy Press, 2101 Constitution Avenue, N.W., Box 285, Washington, D.C. 20055. Call (800) 624-6242 or (202) 334-3313 (in the Washington metropolitan area), or visit the NAP home page at **www.nap.edu.** The full text of this report is available at **www.nap.edu.**

For more information about the Institute of Medicine, visit the IOM home page at: **www.iom.edu.**

THE NATIONAL ACADEMIES

National Academy of Sciences
National Academy of Engineering
Institute of Medicine
National Research Council

The **National Academy of Sciences** is a private, nonprofit, self-perpetuating society of distinguished scholars engaged in scientific and engineering research, dedicated to the furtherance of science and technology and to their use for the general welfare. Upon the authority of the charter granted to it by the Congress in 1863, the Academy has a mandate that requires it to advise the federal government on scientific and technical matters. Dr. Bruce M. Alberts is president of the National Academy of Sciences.

The **National Academy of Engineering** was established in 1964, under the charter of the National Academy of Sciences, as a parallel organization of outstanding engineers. It is autonomous in its administration and in the selection of its members, sharing with the National Academy of Sciences the responsibility for advising the federal government. The National Academy of Engineering also sponsors engineering programs aimed at meeting national needs, encourages education and research, and recognizes the superior achievements of engineers. Dr. William A. Wulf is president of the National Academy of Engineering.

The **Institute of Medicine** was established in 1970 by the National Academy of Sciences to secure the services of eminent members of appropriate professions in the examination of policy matters pertaining to the health of the public. The Institute acts under the responsibility given to the National Academy of Sciences by its congressional charter to be an adviser to the federal government and, upon its own initiative, to identify issues of medical care, research, and education. Dr. Kenneth I. Shine is president of the Institute of Medicine.

The **National Research Council** was organized by the National Academy of Sciences in 1916 to associate the broad community of science and technology with the Academy's purposes of furthering knowledge and advising the federal government. Functioning in accordance with general policies determined by the Academy, the Council has become the principal operating agency of both the National Academy of Sciences and the National Academy of Engineering in providing services to the government, the public, and the scientific and engineering communities. The Council is administered jointly by both Academies and the Institute of Medicine. Dr. Bruce M. Alberts and Dr. William A. Wulf are chairman and vice chairman, respectively, of the National Research Council.

Sandra Millon Underwood, ACS Oncology Nursing Professor, University of Wisconsin School of Nursing, Milwaukee

Frances Visco, President, National Breast Cancer Coalition, Washington, D.C. *(member through April 2001)*

Susan Weiner, President, The Children's Cause, Silver Spring, MD

Study Staff

Hellen Gelband, Study Director

Florence Poillon, Editor

NCPB Staff

Robert Cook-Deegan, Director, National Cancer Policy Board *(through August 2000)*

Roger Herdman, Director, National Cancer Policy Board *(from September 2000)*

Ellen Johnson, Administrator *(through July 2000)*

Nicci T. Dowd, Administrator *(from August 2000)*

Jennifer Cangco, Financial Associate

BACKGROUND PAPER AUTHORS

This summary and the recommendations presented in this report are based on the work of the experts listed below. The background papers they wrote comprise Part 2 of the full report, which is available from the National Academy Press.[1] (Chapter titles are listed on pages 4-5 of this report.)

Lisa Chertkov, M.D., Memorial Sloan-Kettering Cancer Center
Charles S. Cleeland, Ph.D., University of Texas M.D. Anderson Cancer
    Center
David R. Freyer, D.O., DeVos Children's Hospital, Grand Rapids, MI
Sarah Friebert, M.D., Case Western Reserve University, St. Vincent's
    Mercy Children's Hospital, Hospice of the Western Reserve
Joanne M. Hilden, M.D., The Cleveland Clinic Foundation
Bruce P. Himelstein, M.D., University of Pennsylvania School of
    Medicine, Children's Hospital of Philadelphia
Jimmie C. Holland, M.D., Memorial Sloan-Kettering Cancer Center
Javier R. Kane, M.D., University of Texas Health Science Center,
    Christus Santa Rosa Children's Hospital, Christus Santa Rosa
    Hospice
Aaron S. Kesselheim, University of Pennsylvania
Joanne Lynn, M.D., RAND Center to Improve Care of the Dying
Ann O'Mara, R.N., Ph.D., Bethesda, MD
Richard Payne, M.D., Memorial Sloan-Kettering Cancer Center
Joan M. Teno, M.D., M.S., Brown University School of Medicine and
    Department of Community Health

---

[1] *Improving Palliative Care for Cancer*, Kathleen M. Foley and Hellen Gelband, eds., Institute of Medicine. 2001. Washington, D.C.: National Academy Press.

Reviewers

This report has been reviewed in draft form by individuals chosen for their diverse perspectives and technical expertise, in accordance with procedures approved by the NRC's Report Review Committee. The purpose of this independent review is to provide candid and critical comments that will assist the institution in making its published report as sound as possible and to ensure that the report meets institutional standards for objectivity, evidence, and responsiveness to the study charge. The review comments and draft manuscript remain confidential to protect the integrity of the deliberative process. We wish to thank the following individuals for their review of this report:

Susan Dale Block, Dana Farber Cancer Institute
Eduardo Bruera, University of Texas, M.D. Anderson Cancer Center
LaVera M. Crawley, Stanford University Center for Biomedical Ethics
Betty R. Ferrell, City of Hope National Medical Center
Priscilla Kissick, Philadelphia, Pennsylvania
Joseph S. Pagano, University of North Carolina at Chapel Hill
Thomas Smith, Medical College of Virginia
T. Declan Walsh, The Cleveland Clinic Foundation
George Wetherill, Carnegie Institution of Washington

Although the reviewers listed above have provided many constructive comments and suggestions, they were not asked to endorse the conclusions or recommendations nor did they see the final draft of the report before its release. The review of this report was overseen by Harold Sox of the Dartmouth-Hitchcock Medical Center, appointed by the NRC's Report Review Committee, who was responsible for making certain that an independent examination of this report was carried out in accordance with institutional procedures and that all review comments were carefully considered. Responsibility for the final content of this report rests entirely with the National Cancer Policy Board, the Institute of Medicine, and the National Research Council.

Preface

It is innately human to comfort and provide care to those suffering from cancer, particularly those close to death. Yet what seems self-evident at an individual, personal level has, by and large, not guided policy at the level of institutions in this country. There is no argument that palliative care should be integrated into cancer care from diagnosis to death. But significant barriers—attitudinal, behavioral, economic, educational, and legal—still limit access to care for a large proportion of those dying from cancer, and in spite of tremendous scientific opportunities for medical progress against all the major symptoms associated with cancer and cancer death, public research institutions have not responded. In accepting a single-minded focus on research toward cure, we have inadvertently devalued the critical need to care for and support patients with advanced disease, and their families.

This report builds on and takes forward an agenda set out by the 1997 IOM report *Approaching Death: Improving Care at the End of Life*, which came at a time when leaders in palliative care and related fields had already begun to air issues surrounding care of the dying. That report identified significant gaps in knowledge about care at the end of life and the need for serious attention from biomedical, social science, and health services researchers. Most importantly, it recognized that the impediments to good care could be identified and potentially remedied. The report itself catalyzed further public involvement in specific initiatives—mostly pilot and demonstration projects and programs funded by the nonprofit foundation community, which are now coming to fruition.

There are no villains in this piece but ourselves and our culture. Public institutions and policymakers reflect dominant societal values that still deny dying and death. Although it does occur, change to improve care of the suffering and dying is slow and conflicted with the tension between cure and care. This report encourages continued innovation and collaboration of foundations and others, but focuses on ways in which the government can embrace opportunities to improve existing palliative care, make access to it equitable for all, and help realize better palliative interventions by making research funds more available.

It is a truism that death—not just our own—affects all of us, even if it is a topic most people do not want to contemplate for long. Death is inevitable, but severe suffering is not. Willpower and determination will be required, but it is time to move our public institutions toward policies that emphasize the importance of improving palliative care for those who want and need it. This report identifies the special needs of cancer patients and the importance of the clinical and research establishment involved in cancer care to take a leadership role in modeling the best quality care from diagnosis to death for all Americans.

Kathleen M. Foley, M.D.
Director, Project on Death in America, The Open Society

Contents

TABLES AND BOXES

Tables

Boxes

Summary

INTRODUCTION

The last half-century produced substantial advances in the treatment and early detection of a few types of cancer and at least modest gains in many others. Yet the reality is that at the beginning of the twenty-first century, half of all patients diagnosed with cancer will die of their disease within a few years. This translates into more than half a million people each year in the United States, and the annual toll will grow as the population ages and more people survive to get cancer over the coming decades.

The imperative in cancer research and treatment has been, understandably, an almost single-minded focus on attempts to cure every patient at every stage of disease. Recognition of the importance of symptom control and other aspects of palliative care from diagnosis through the dying process has been growing, however, and has reached the national health care agenda through the efforts of prominent bodies such as the President's Cancer Panel, the Medicare Payment Advisory Commission, the Institute of Medicine (IOM), and major health care foundations. All conclude that patients should not have to choose between treatment with curative intent *or* comfort care. There is a need for both, in varying degrees, throughout the course of cancer, whether the eventual outcome is long-term survival or death.

The goal is to maintain the best possible quality of life, allowing cancer patients the freedom to choose whatever treatments they so wish throughout the course of the disease, while also meeting the needs of patients with

1

advanced disease through adequate symptom control. This goal is not met for most cancer patients in the United States today. We have words for "survivors" and those in active treatment, but even today, those with advanced disease who are not in active treatment and who are dying are nameless and faceless without a priority.

For at least half of those dying from cancer—most of them elderly and many vulnerable—death entails a spectrum of symptoms, including pain, labored breathing, distress, nausea, confusion and other physical and psychological conditions that go untreated or undertreated and vastly diminish the quality of their remaining days (Donnelly and Walsh, 1995; Phillips et al., 2000). The patient is not the only one who suffers during the dying process. The impact on families and caregivers is still poorly documented, but evidence has begun to be collected demonstrating a heavy and mostly unrelieved emotional and financial burden (Emanuel et al., 2000b). This cannot be ignored within the context of caring for people who are terminally ill.

A major problem in palliative care is the underrecognition, underdiagnosis, and thus undertreatment of patients with significant distress, ranging from existential anguish to anxiety and depression. This situation continues to exist despite the fact that when dying patients themselves have been asked their primary concerns about their care, three of their five concerns were psychosocial: (1) no prolongation of dying; (2) maintaining a sense of control; and (3) relieving burdens (conflicts) and strengthening ties (Singer et al., 1999).

All this is true at the same time that one-quarter of Medicare dollars are spent in the last year of life, and half of that is spent in the last month of life. Living with, and eventually dying from, a chronic illness runs up substantial costs for patient, family, and society, and costs for those dying from cancer are about 20 percent higher than average costs (Hogan et al., 2000). Dying patients are sick, dependent, changing, and needy. Most likely, high costs would be acceptable if patients and families were satisfied with the care provided for those with advanced disease, but few can count on being satisfied. In short, our society is spending a great deal and not getting what dying cancer patients need.

The current inadequacy of palliative and end-of-life care springs not from a single cause or sector of society, but from institutional and economic barriers, lack of information about what can be achieved, lack of training and education of health care professionals, and minuscule public sector investments in research to improve the situation. This is not to suggest that there is no ongoing research on relevant questions or training programs— there are—but the efforts are not coordinated, and there is no locus for these activities in any federal agency. What has resulted is underfunding, a lack of appropriate training, and a lack of research leadership, with no sustained programs for developing and disseminating palliative treatments. Despite the enormous health care expenditures for the dying, less than 1 percent of the National Cancer Institute (NCI) budget is spent on any aspect of symptom control, palliative care, or end-of-life research or training.

WHAT IS PALLIATIVE CARE?

The World Health Organization (WHO) defines palliative care in cancer as the "active total care of patients whose disease is not responsive to curative treatment." The definition is extended in an important way with the statement, "Many aspects of palliative care are also applicable earlier in the course of the illness, in conjunction with anticancer treatment" (WHO, 1990). Palliative care focuses on addressing the control of pain and other symptoms, as well as psychological, social, and spiritual distress. In its recommendation to member governments, WHO states that any national cancer control program should address the needs of its citizens for palliative care. This National Cancer Policy Board report adopts the WHO definition and position, focusing on the importance of palliative care beginning at the time of a cancer diagnosis and increasing in amount and intensity throughout the course of a patient's illness, until death.

In a practical sense, six major skill sets comprise complete palliative care:

1. communication,
2. decisionmaking,
3. management of complications of treatment and the disease,
4. symptom control,
5. psychosocial care of patient and family, and
6. care of the dying.

Some of these skills—communication, decisionmaking, psychosocial care of patient and family—are important throughout the trajectory of illness. Others emerge and recede in importance at different times. Treatment and prevention of complications caused by primary cancer treatments are generally episodic, though some require long-term management. Disease complications may require a variety of interventions (including surgery and radiation) that, for many, do not fit neatly into a palliative care definition. The need for symptom control unrelated to treatment generally increases as a person approaches death, but at least for some patients, it begins much earlier. Symptom control is never, however, a substitute for primary cancer care that is desired by a patient.

INTENT OF THIS REPORT

The National Cancer Policy Board (NCPB) recognized that excellent palliative care is possible but is not being delivered to a large number of those living with and dying from cancer. In its report *Ensuring Quality Cancer Care* (IOM, 1999) one of the Board's recommendations was: "Ensure quality of care at the end of life, in particular, the management of cancer-related pain and timely referral to palliative and hospice care."

The current report delves into and expands on that mandate, addressing not only what can be done for people now nearing the end of life, but also setting a course for the development of better treatments and better ways of delivering and paying for them. This report also takes forward the agenda outlined in an influential 1997 IOM report *Approaching Death: Improving Care at the End of Life*, the first comprehensive, evidence-based, national report on these issues, which stimulated widespread interest and progress in some aspects of care for the dying. With the 1997 and 1999 reports as backdrop, the current effort focuses on specific areas in which the Board believes action still has to be catalyzed.

To accomplish this, eight papers were commissioned, which comprise Part II of the full report. This stand-alone summary, which appears as Chaper 1 of the full report, draws on these papers and other sources, and ends with a set of broad-based recommendations supported by the evidence supplied in the commissioned papers. The papers themselves, which appear in the full report, should be consulted for many more suggestions of specific activities and actions to be considered. The titles and authors of the chapters, which comprise Part II of the full report, follow:

- *Chapter 2: Reliable, High-Quality, Efficient End-of-Life Care for Cancer Patients: Economic Issues and Barriers, Joanne Lynn and Ann O'Mara*
- *Chapter 3: Quality of Life and Quality Indicators for End-of-Life Cancer Care: Hope for the Best, Yet Prepare for the Worst, Joan M. Teno*
- *Chapter 4: The Current State of Patient and Family Information About End-of-Life Care, Aaron S. Kesselheim*
- *Chapter 5: Palliative Care for African Americans and Other Vulnerable Populations: Access and Quality Issues, Richard Payne*
- *Chapter 6: End-of-Life Care: Special Issues in Pediatric Oncology, Joanne M. Hilden, Bruce P. Himelstein, David R. Freyer, Sarah Friebert, and Javier R. Kane*
- *Chapter 7: Clinical Practice Guidelines for the Management of Psychosocial and Physical Symptoms of Cancer, Jimmie C. Holland and Lisa Chertkov*

- *Chapter 8: Cross-Cutting Research Issues: A Research Agenda for Reducing Distress of Patients with Cancer, Charles S. Cleeland*
- *Chapter 9: Professional Education in Palliative and End-of-Life Care for Physicians, Nurses, and Social Workers, Hellen Gelband*

The report focuses exclusively on deaths from cancer, despite the fact that the number of people in the United States dying from other chronic diseases exceeds the number dying from cancer. Many of the issues raised and recommendations made in the report should benefit people dying from all these conditions, and it is not the NCPB's intent to divert attention from the many people dying from congestive heart failure, kidney disease, or other chronic diseases. There is a logic, however, to looking at cancer deaths alone, aside from the obvious point that this report is a product of the National Cancer Policy Board.

Cancer has been the "prototype" disease for organizing end-of-life care for several reasons: it has a more predictable trajectory from the point at which cure becomes unlikely until death than other chronic diseases; the most frequent and distressing symptoms are similar for many forms of cancer; there is a nationwide infrastructure of cancer centers carrying on cancer research, treating a significant minority of patients, and influencing the practice of oncology across the country; and the most generously funded of the National Institutes of Health (NIH)—NCI, approaching $4 billion in 2001—is focused on cancer.

The report points out deficiencies in the way patients with advanced cancer are treated, but this does not signify that oncology is behind other medical disciplines in palliative care in general or in care for dying patients. In fact, the cancer establishment has played a leading role in the area of pain management, using the cancer patient with pain as a model for other conditions and developing national guidelines and educational initiatives. Hospice care also developed around the needs of advanced cancer patients in close association with the cancer establishment. With that head start, cancer professionals are poised to take the lead in other areas of symptom control and the organization and delivery of excellent palliative care.

BARRIERS TO EXCELLENT PALLIATIVE AND END-OF-LIFE CARE

Barriers throughout the health care and medical research systems stand in the way of many people receiving effective palliative care where and when they need it. These barriers include

- the separation of palliative and hospice care from potentially life-prolonging treatment within the health care system, which is both influenced by and affects reimbursement policy;

- inadequate training of health care personnel in symptom management and other palliative care skills;
- inadequate standards of care and lack of accountability in caring for dying patients;
- disparities in care, even when available, for African Americans and other ethnic and socioeconomic segments of the population;
- lack of information resources for the public dealing with palliative and end-of-life care;
- lack of reliable data on the quality of life and the quality of care of patients dying from cancer (as well as other chronic diseases) and lack of accountability for providing excellent end-of-life care within the health care system; and
- low level of public sector investment in palliative and end-of-life care research and training.

Separation of Palliative and Hospice Care Within the Health Care System

A major barrier to adequate palliative care has been the institutionalization of a system that focuses on *either* active therapy *or* palliative or hospice care and does not allow the appropriate interface between these two approaches. In Part II of the full report, Lynn and O'Mara (Chapter 2) describe the ways in which this split is reinforced by the rules governing hospice care under the Medicare program, the largest payer of care for dying Americans. In addition, Holland and Chertkov (Chapter 7) describe the lack of attention to psychosocial, existential, and spiritual needs even when palliative care is available, and Payne (Chapter 5) describes the unequal access and even poorer treatment often afforded African Americans and other special population groups.

Hospice is the most substantial innovation to serve dying Americans, and for most, it is paid for by the Medicare hospice benefit (using a per diem rate), which was created in 1982. Hospice services—which are predominantly home based—include many elements that are not typically part of Medicare coverage (e.g., an interdisciplinary team, care planning, personal care nursing, family and patient teaching and support, chaplaincy, medication [with a small copayment], medical equipment and supplies, counseling, symptomatic treatment, bereavement support). However, Medicare allows hospice enrollment only for patients with a "prognosis of less than six months" and it is only with difficulty that hospices deal with documentation requirements for longer stays. These requirements ensure that hospice enrollment is seen as a decision to pursue a death-accepting course, which is an obvious deterrent for many patients. Furthermore, hospices are prohibited from offering any of their services to patients who are not formally enrolled, but who might benefit from some aspects of hospice care.

In recent years, more than 60 percent of patients who have enrolled in the Medicare hospice benefit have had cancer, and more than half of all dying cancer patients have used some hospice services (Hogan et al., 2000). The creation of the Medicare benefit was a major step forward, but its strict and limiting rules have led to inappropriately short stays of patients in hospice care, depriving them of the full application of palliative care in the final days of their lives.

The interface of hospice services and nursing home care is also unsettled. Nursing home stays are reimbursed by Medicare for only a minority of patients, but for these patients, Medicare reimbursement is high enough that they are unlikely to be offered the opportunity to enroll in hospice (only either skilled nursing home care or hospice can be in effect at one time). Since most nursing home stays do not qualify for Medicare payment, patients in nursing homes are often eligible for hospice services, but administrative complications deter enrollment for a large proportion of them.

The hospice requirement of a "six-month" prognosis has never been defined and is the source of trouble. Is the "just barely qualified" patient simply "more likely than not" to die within six months, or should that patient be "virtually certain to die"? This may seem like an arcane issue, but the population of everyone who is more likely than not to die within six months is *two to three orders of magnitude* (100 to 1,000 times) larger than the population that is virtually certain to die. The uncertainty of definition affects the willingness of hospices to accept patients who might stabilize and live a long time. Well-publicized fraud investigations for long-stay hospice patients (e.g., Lagnado, 2000, in the *Wall Street Journal*) have increased the chances that these patients, who are chronically ill and have benefited from hospice care, are likely to be discharged.

A number of other issues that affect access to and use of hospice services cause concern for patients and hospice providers. Hospices have significant latitude in deciding what services to offer, and they can vary tremendously, so patients are faced with selecting among them to find the best fit. Hospices are bedeviled with short stays, which have gotten shorter in recent years (from an average of 90 days in 1990 [Christakis and Escarce, 1996] to 48 days in 1999 [National Hospice and Palliative Care Organization, 2001]). No reliable research has yet sorted out the sources of increasingly short stays, but the financial impact on hospices has been substantial. The first day or two and the last few days in hospice are always costly. When these days come close together, there can be too few "stable" days with lower costs to offset losses on the "expensive days."

Hospices struggle with a plethora of developments in palliative care.

Twenty years ago, it was not much of an exaggeration to claim that the hospice physician could do most everything with little more than cheap opioid medications, steroids, diuretics, and antibiotics. Now, there are more technologically advanced interventions, more expensive medications, more use of radiation or surgery, and so on—and additional costs of keeping hospice staff trained in their use—yet the Medicare hospice payment is a fixed amount per day. Some hospice programs rely on philanthropic donations to cover expensive interventions that they would not otherwise be able to offer.

Not everyone dying of cancer is covered by Medicare. The special case of children, analyzed by Hilden and colleagues (Chapter 6 in the full report), demonstrates severe problems in securing and being paid for adequate palliative care through private insurers. Holland and Chertkov (Chapter 7 in the full report) add that reimbursement for professional psychosocial care is poor to absent even in major cancer centers and is often excluded from medical and behavioral health contracts.

Some small-scale innovative demonstration projects are under way to test new ways of providing and paying for good palliative care throughout the course of fatal illness (e.g., see Box 1), but it is too soon to recommend a comprehensive set of changes (particularly for Medicare) without further experience, experimentation, and evaluation. A period of innovation, with thoughtful evaluation and learning, is needed in order to shape the care system and payment arrangements that would better serve cancer patients coming to the end of life.

Inadequate Training of Health Care Personnel

Most U.S. physicians—oncologists, other specialists, and generalists alike—are not prepared by education or experience to satisfy the palliative care needs of dying cancer patients or even to help them get needed services from other providers (Emanuel, 2000). The same holds for the other mainstays of end-of-life care: nurses and social workers. In a review of the education and training of professionals, in Part II of the full report, Gelband (Chapter 9) reports that this finding is consistent with the lack of funding for end-of-life or palliative care educational initiatives, which has begun to change only recently. Needs in training and education were covered in depth in the IOM (1997) report *Approaching Death*, and some of the new programs have taken root as a result of that report. Even in 2000, however, the programs were small and funded largely by private grant-making organizations, with little contribution by the federal government. Holland and Chertkov (Chapter 7) attribute much of the difficulty that patients find in getting adequate treatment to the fact that there are no training standards to prepare physicians to identify patients with distress, nor are there stan-

**Box 1
Promoting Excellence in End-of-Life Care—
The Robert Wood Johnson Foundation**

Typically, patients with incurable cancers do not receive palliative care in the form of hospice until all life-prolonging options have been exhausted, often within just two weeks of death. As part of its "Promoting Excellence in End-of-Life Care" program, the Robert Wood Johnson Foundation began, in 1999, funding three-year demonstration projects at four cancer centers around the country to test innovative, integrated models of palliative and cancer care. The projects, located in Michigan, New Hampshire, Ohio, and California, are independent and are organized differently, but with common themes. Using approaches designed to fit within their particular health systems, each project is striving to incorporate palliative care within the continuum of cancer treatment from diagnosis through the trajectory of illness, extending to bereavement support for patients' families. Interdisciplinary teams, which may include physicians, nurses, social workers, and pastoral care providers, respond to the needs of patients and families. Emphasis is accorded communication, advance care planning, symptom management, and coordination of medical and support services.

Disease-modifying therapy is provided, including available NCI clinical trials. Patients with advanced cancer, or those whose cancers are deemed incurable at onset, are eligible for enrollment in these demonstrations. Project evaluation focuses on the feasibility and acceptability of these new models to patients, their families, and the collaborating local health systems. Outcome measures include clinical parameters of longevity, symptom frequency and severity, patient-family satisfaction, and quality of life. Utilization of resources, including hospitalizations, intensive care unit admissions, use of hospice services, and hospice lengths of stay, are also being studied.

A key to all of the programs is laying out options for care at an earlier stage of illness than usually occurs. Particularly important is avoiding the "terrible choice" that the health care system now imposes between potentially life-prolonging treatment and pure palliative care ("active" treatment versus "hospice") and to smooth the transition from one to the other when necessary. Brief descriptions of the programs and some early results are presented here.

1. The Palliative Care Program—University of Michigan Comprehensive Cancer Center

Researchers at the University of Michigan's Comprehensive Cancer Center, in conjunction with Hospice of Michigan, are integrating hospice services into the care of patients with advanced breast, prostate, or lung cancer or advanced congestive heart failure, while potentially life-prolonging treatment continues. They are conducting a randomized trial that follows on a pilot study involving patients with advanced prostate cancer, which found improvements in patient comfort and satisfaction when palliative care was provided concomitant with disease-modifying treatments.

According to Dr. Kenneth J. Pienta, a principal investigator for the project, "Within this new system, the patient and family can appropriately begin the process of transition and we can provide an opportunity for patients and families to grow through the end of life."

box continued on next page

In the first year, 84 patients enrolled in the trial. In this early group, no overall difference is seen in standard quality-of-life measures two months after enrollment, but for those who functional status was poorer to begin with (Karnofsky score d70), the program appears to have improved quality of life in the intervention group compared with the usual care group, with the suggestion of a greater effect over time.

2. Project ENABLE: Educate, Nurture, Advise, Before Life Ends— Dartmouth-Hitchcock Medical Center

The Dartmouth-Hitchcock Medical Center's ENABLE Project team has moved high-quality end-of-life care into New Hampshire's regional cancer center and beyond, into three rural communities. The ENABLE team assesses patients' needs and provides continuous palliative care throughout the course of cancer care. Patient education is a priority. The team travels to each town with a unique educational seminar, "Charting Your Course: A Whole Person's Approach to Living with Cancer," empowering cancer patients and their families to better navigate the health care system, engage in advanced care planning, and extending support to those confronting issues of life completion and closure. The goal is to help people retain control of their lives and key decisions.

Following diagnosis, a palliative care coordinator works with patients and families to develop a care plan, stressing continuity of care during the course of the illness. Each of the three communities has a palliative care team, consisting of a pain management specialist, a psychiatrist or psychologist, a hospice or home health liaison, a social worker or case manager, and a pastoral caregiver. Each team tailors its work to the specific health care system in the community.

"Project ENABLE will allow us to demonstrate that, regardless of geographic location, cultural identification, or clinical sophistication, patients need not be abandoned when a cure for their disease seems no longer possible," said E. Robert Greenberg, M.D., principal investigator for the project.

One early indication of the program's success at merging the cultures of hospice and oncology treatment is the commitment shown by six staff oncologists in sitting for—and passing—the certification exam in palliative medicine.

3. Project Safe Conduct—Ireland Cancer Center, Case Western Reserve University

Case Western Reserve University Hospitals of Cleveland has literally invited the palliative team into the Ireland Cancer Center. The Project Safe Conduct team's office is in the same building, and each member of the team wears an Ireland Cancer Center nametag. The team attends staff orientations and meets regularly with the therapeutic staff. Physician acceptance of the program is high, and patients have been recruited to the program faster than anticipated. This collaboration between the cancer center, Hospice of the Western Reserve, and Case Western Reserve University creates a system that allows patients to receive life-prolonging care—including experimental therapy protocols—integrated with palliative care. In Project Safe Conduct, patients and families are guided through the labyrinth of available treatments and services, emphasizing state-of-the-art symptom management as well as psychosocial and spiritual support.

Early results are encouraging. In the first year, 133 patients were enrolled, of whom 40 percent were members of ethnic or racial minorities. Pain assessment has been documented in 100 percent of Safe Conduct patients, compared to a historical control of just 3 percent. Quality-of-life scores remained steady or improved in Safe Conduct patients, despite concomitant decline in functional status. At baseline, only 13 percent of the center's patients were served by hospice and for an average of just 3 days before death. Now, only 18 months into the Safe Conduct Project, more than 80 percent of Ireland's patients have the benefits of hospice care, achieving an average length of stay of 18 days.

As part of the effort, Project Safe Conduct is also developing innovative palliative care curricula for the Case Western Reserve Schools of Medicine and Nursing, as well as postgraduate training for specialists in oncology.

4. Improvements in End-of-Life Care for Selected Populations—University of California-Davis Cancer Center

Researchers at the University of California-Davis (UC Davis) Medical Center and the West Coast Center for Palliative Education, Sacramento, California, have developed the Simultaneous Care project to extend palliative care to patients undergoing active, anticancer treatments (who would otherwise be ineligible for hospice care). In Simultaneous Care, palliative care staff work together with clinical oncologists to serve patients with advanced cancer, including those participating in experimental treatment protocols. In early results, quality of life as measured by the FACT (Functional Assessment of Cancer Therapy) shows a clear trend toward improvement for Simultaneous Care patients compared to patients receiving best customary care. There has also been a greater adherence to chemotherapy protocols for Simultaneous Care patients, a higher percentage of referrals to hospice, and improved length of stays in hospice. Finally, preliminary data suggest that the distress experienced by primary caregivers may be reduced, both during the illness and after the patient's death.

In another aspect of this project, some of California's hardest-to-serve populations are also being reached. The program expands and improves the level of palliative care available to people in three isolated, rural areas—Colusa, Tuolumne, and Plumas Counties—as well as the state women's prison population. According to the project's principal investigator, Dr. Frederick J. Meyers, although they are dissimilar in many ways, each of the targeted populations lacks access to palliative or hospice care.

In this project, palliative care experts have trained teams of health providers to work in the rural counties and to use teleconferencing links to UC Davis physicians for immediate assistance in the care of dying patients. Using remote television, UC Davis physicians consult with patients and offer suggestions for care. In a third component of the project, staff are working with California Department of Corrections and health care teams in the women's prison to offer palliative care training and begin development of a prison hospice program to serve inmates who are dying.

dards of competence for those who provide psychosocial and spiritual services at the end of life.

Most new physicians leave medical school and residency programs with little training or experience in caring for dying patients. In most cases, a few lectures are folded into other courses (in many cases in psychiatry and behavioral sciences, ethics, or the humanities). A few schools offer full-length courses on palliative care, but they are nearly all electives. Contact with dying patients, particularly for undergraduate medical students, if any, is limited.

Nurses are expected to provide physical, emotional, spiritual, and practical care for patients in every phase of life. They spend more time with patients near the end of life than do any other health professionals. Yet like physicians, most nurses in the United States do not receive the training and practical experience they need to carry out these duties in the best fashion. The nursing curriculum has been less studied than the medical curriculum, but this has been changing, particularly in response to debates about assisted suicide and euthanasia (Ferrell et al., 2000).

Social workers are central to counseling, case management, and advocacy services for the dying and for bereaved families. With their focus on the psychosocial aspects of the dying process, they work not only with patients but with those around them in making decisions about treatment options, marshaling resources, helping families cope with terminal illness and death of a relative, and generally encouraging the best quality of life for all concerned. Just as nursing and medicine have begun to do, the social work profession has been examining its education process for preparing practitioners to care for dying patients and their families. Efforts to improve undergraduate- and master's-level social work training in this area are just getting under way in the United States, in comparison to the more mature field in Canada and England and in comparison to medical and nursing education (Christ and Sormanti, 1999).

In medicine, nursing, and social work, the following are needed:

- faculty development,
- educational materials and curriculum development,
- coordination among training programs for the variety of professionals involved in the care of dying patients,
- guidelines for residency programs and increased palliative and end-of-life content in licensing and certifying examinations, and
- improving the research base for palliative care education.

Inadequate Standards of Care and Lack of Accountability in Caring for Dying Patients

Practice Guidelines

The process of developing standards of care for patients at the end of life is under way, but still at an early stage. In Part II of the full report, Holland and Chertkov (Chapter 7) review the status of practice guidelines for care at the end of life, including both physical and psychosocial components (Table 1). The one aspect for which evidence-based guidelines for end-of-life care do exist is pain management. In addition to general pain management guidelines (the Agency for Healthcare Research and Quality [AHRQ] and the National Comprehensive Cancer Network [NCCN]), guidelines specifically for pain control at the end of life have been developed. Work is progressing on guidelines for some other common symptoms. NCCN guidelines exist for a variety of psychosocial conditions— distress, delirium, depression, anxiety, personality disorders, social problems, and spiritual and religious issues—but they are general and have to be modified for dying patients (a process that is under way through NCCN). A guideline for fatigue is in the same state, and one for nausea and vomiting has been developed for treatment-related symptoms, but not for end-of-life symptoms. No guidelines exist for managing dyspnea, a frequent and distressing symptom.

Various groups are working toward guidelines in these areas (despite, in many cases, a lack of evidence forcing reliance on consensus), but plans for validation and field testing are probably years off for most of them.

Accountability: Quality Indicators

It is not enough to define the best treatments and develop models of excellent palliative and end-of-life care, or even to educate health care providers about what works and what doesn't, although these are all necessary steps. What is important is that dying patients, in the variety of health care settings in which they receive care, actually get the best treatments. The NCPB report *Ensuring Quality Cancer Care* (IOM, 1999) outlined a vision for the development of "indicators" to cover the spectrum of cancer care—including the dying process—that could be used to hold health care providers, institutions, and health plans accountable for the quality of care given.

As Teno demonstrates in Chapter 3 of the full report, we are not close to meeting this mandate for care at the end of life, either for cancer or for other conditions (Table 2). Research and demonstration programs will be needed before even a preliminary set of satisfactory indicators can be devel-

TABLE 1 Clinical Practice Guidelines for End-of-Life Care: Status, Source, and Further Development Needed

Symptom	Status	Source	Further Development
Overall end-of-life care	NCCN Practice Guidelines (pending) (NCCN, 2001)	Evidence, consensus, or combination	Pilot testing; modify for end-of-life care
Doctor-patient communication	NCCN Practice Guidelines: breaking bad news (pending) (NCCN, 2001)	Evidence, consensus, or combination	Pilot testing; modify for end-of-life care
Distress	NCCN Practice Guidelines: ambulatory care Definition—Psychosocial, existential or spiritual (NCCN, 1999)		Algorithm for recognition and referral; modify for end-of-life care
Delirium	APA Practice Guidelines: physically healthy (APA, 2000)	Evidence, consensus, or combination	Modify for medically ill and end-of-life care
	NCCN Practice Guidelines: ambulatory care (NCCN, 1999)	Evidence, consensus, or combination	Modify for end-of-life care; pilot test
Depressive disorders	APA Practice Guidelines: physically healthy (APA, 2000)	Evidence, consensus, or combination	Modify for end-of-life care
	NCCN Practice Guidelines: ambulatory care (NCCN, 1999)	Evidence, consensus, or combination	Modify for end-of-life care; pilot test

TABLE 1 Continued

Symptom	Status	Source	Further Development
Anxiety disorders	APA Practice Guidelines: panic disorder in healthy patients (APA, 2000)	Evidence, consensus, or combination	Modify for medically ill/ end-of-life care
	NCCN Practice Guidelines: ambulatory care (NCCN, 1999)	Evidence, consensus, or combination	Modify for end-of-life care; pilot test
Personality disorders	APA Practice Guidelines (APA, 2000)	Evidence, consensus, or combination	Modify for medically ill and end-of-life care
	NCCN Practice Guidelines: ambulatory care (NCCN, 1999)	Evidence, consensus, or combination	Modify for end-of-life care; pilot test
Social problems: practical or psychosocial	NCCN Guidelines for Social Work Services: Ambulatory (NCCN, 1999)	Evidence, consensus, or combination	Modify for end-of-life care; pilot test
Spiritual or religious problems	NCCN Guidelines for Clergy/ Pastoral Counselors: ambulatory (NCCN, 1999)	Evidence, consensus, or combination	Modify for end-of-life care; pilot test
Pain	AHCPR Guidelines (AHCPR, 1994)	Evidence, consensus, or combination	Modify for end-of-life care
	APS Guidelines (APS, 1995)	Evidence, consensus, or combination	Dissemination and implementation
	WHO Pain Management (WHO, 1996)	Evidence, consensus, or combination	Compliance and implementation

continued on next page

TABLE 1 Continued

Symptom	Status	Source	Further Development
	NCCN Guidelines (NCCN, 1999)	Evidence, consensus, or combination	Modify for end-of-life care; pilot test; dissemination and compliance
Fatigue	NCCN Practice Guidelines: guidelines for anemia-related fatigue management (NCCN, 1999)	Evidence, consensus, or combination	Modify for end-of-life care; pilot test
Nausea and vomiting	NCCN anti-emesis (for treatment-related nausea and vomiting) (NCCN, 1997)	Evidence, consensus, or combination	Modify for end-of-life care; pilot test
Dyspnea	Descriptive guides to care (Ahmedzai, 1998)	Literature	Develop guidelines; pilot test

NOTE: APA = American Psychiatric Association; APS = American Pain Society; AHCPR = Agency for Health Care Policy and Research; NCCN = National Comprehensive Cancer Network

oped. The focus of early work will be on the development and validation of measurement tools based on administrative data, medical records, and interviews with patients, family members, and health care providers. These instruments must be developed and adapted for different cultures and ethnicities.

Quality indicators are needed for two main purposes: accountability (external use by regulators, health care purchasers, or consumers) and quality improvement (internal use for the purpose of monitoring or continuous quality improvement). The same types of indicators may serve both purposes, but for some aspects, they may have to be different.

At this early stage in development, there is a strong evidence base to support the use of quality indicators for pain management for the purpose of accountability, and in fact, a standard (not specific to end-of-life care or cancer) has just taken effect through the Joint Commission on Accreditation of Healthcare Organizations (JCAHO), requiring all participating hospitals to demonstrate that they adequately monitor and manage the pain of

TABLE 2 Status of Quality Indicator Development for End-of-Life Care

Domain	Proposed Indicators	Readiness
Pain	Frequency and severity of pain from Minimum Data Set	Proposed indicators require validation, but can be measured for all hospitalized cancer patients Major limitation: captures only health care provider perspective
	Patient and family perspective on pain management	Instruments available (e.g., from American Pain Society or Toolkit of Instruments to Measure End-of-Life Care)
Satisfaction	Measures of patient satisfaction, based on patient or surrogate responses New instruments include some questions relevant to people dying from cancer	New instruments have undergone reliability and validity testing. Additional questions are specific for cancer (e.g., whether patients are informed of recommended treatments, access to high-quality clinical trials) and incorporation into ongoing data collection efforts
Shared Decisionmaking	Questions from Toolkit of Instruments to Measure End-of-Life Care	Reliability and validity testing completed Examination of responsiveness not complete
Coordination and Continuity of Care	No indicators yet available	

patients (JCAHO, 2000). However, more basic research and demonstration projects are needed to develop indicators for managing other common symptoms (e.g., emotional distress and depression, fatigue, gastrointestinal symptoms). An important aspect of demonstration and validation is monitoring for potential unintended consequences (e.g., patients are sedated contrary to their preferences to improve accountability statistics).

Besides the domain of symptom management, four other domains should be considered for early development and implementation of accountability measures: (1) patient satisfaction, (2) shared decisionmaking, (3) coordination, and (4) continuity of care. In each of these domains, indicators must validly represent the perceptions of the dying person and family members. This means investing in new survey methods that are patient centered and include questions that get at unmet needs.

Shared decisionmaking has been increasingly recognized as a key aspect throughout the continuum of care. Although the focus of research has been on resuscitation decisions, the most important decision for the majority of cancer patients is the one to stop active treatment, but there is little research that examines this decision.

Beyond those mentioned, there is debate over which other domains are important in the care of the dying. Various conceptual models have been proposed to examine the quality of end-of-life care, with different emphases. Research is now needed to examine the correlations among structures of the health care system, processes of care, and important outcomes to identify the most fruitful areas for developing new quality measures.

Ongoing national data collection efforts include little information to describe the quality of care of dying persons and their families. An occasional survey, the National Mortality Followback Survey (NMFBS), has collected information on access to care and functional status, but not on important domains that are central to the quality of care of the dying. A redesigned NMFBS could collect information on key domains to describe the quality of care for patients who died based on the perspective of the bereaved family member. There are no current plans for further iterations of the NMFBS, however.

Two national data collection systems warrant consideration for development of quality indicators: Medicare claims files and the Nursing Home Minimum Data Set (MDS). The NCPB has recommended previously that hospice enrollment and length of stay be examined as quality indicators (IOM, 1999). From a national perspective, the only source of that information is Medicare claims data. Other indicators based on administrative data have also been proposed. Work to develop and validate these indicators using claims data is still to be done.

The second national data collection effort is the MDS, which routinely collects extensive information on every nursing home resident in the United States. Nursing homes increasingly are providing end-of-life care for frail and older Americans. In 1998, an estimated 10 percent of cancer patients died in a nursing home. The Health Care Financing Administration (HCFA) is now embarking on a national program of examining nursing home quality performance. There are important lessons to be learned from the MDS, including concerns about the institutional response burden in implementing data collection and the potential for unintended consequences. In the nursing home setting, a concern is that quality indicators have been developed for the majority of nursing home residents (who are not dying imminently) where the main goals of care are to restore function, yet the same indicators will be applied to those who are dying. For example, the rates of dehydration and weight loss are now among the core quality indicators for nursing homes. With increased scrutiny of these indicators, there is concern that unintended consequences for the dying might include increased use of feeding tubes, which could be contrary to patient preferences.

Disparities in End-of-Life Care for Minority Groups

Cancer statistics for certain minority groups in the United States reveal substantial inequalities in health outcomes. African Americans represent the largest minority population, and the one for which there is the best documentation of unequal access to, and quality of, care. Cancer incidence and mortality rates are significantly higher, and survival rates significantly lower, for African Americans than for whites in the United States. African Americans are also underrepresented in the use of hospice care. In recent years, only 5-7 percent of hospice patients have been African Americans, even though they make up about 14 percent of the total population. In Chapter 5 of the full report, Payne describes the historical, cultural, and economic determinants of this pattern of underutilization of palliative and end-of-life care in the African-American population, which can be taken as a model for other medically underserved and vulnerable populations that are less well studied. Bias (conscious and unconscious) of health care providers, lack of economic access for many African-American and other minority group members, and a wide range of cultural factors place minority groups at a disadvantage in getting adequate palliative care.

Unequal treatment in the U.S. health care system has deep roots in the African-American community. The health care system, along with many other societal institutions, lacks credibility with many African Americans because of past abuses, which are commonly known: slavery, medical experimentation, Jim Crow laws, and so forth. Denial of death (even in the face of terminal illness) is seen—if unconsciously—as fighting back against past injustice; whereas accepting palliative care is viewed as giving up on care that the majority might receive.

Even when palliative care is wanted and needed, however, it may not be available. Hospice care may not be available in poor, inner-city areas, which are generally underserved for health care. A stark example comes from a recent study demonstrating that pharmacies in predominantly non-white communities do not stock opioids at all or have inadequate stocks (Morrison et al., 2000). In an accompanying editorial, the story is recounted of an elderly woman with unrelieved bone pain from metastatic cancer, whose daughter was unable to buy a prescribed morphine-based drug in any local pharmacy (Freeman and Payne, 2000). This is just an example of inequities that pervade the provision of palliative care for minority populations.

There is an urgent need for palliative care units in inner-city hospitals, which involves not only providing facilities, but training teams of providers to staff these units. Even more fundamental, research is required to understand the needs and preferences of African Americans and other minorities for end-of-life care and to elucidate the health policy and financial barriers that leave these groups with inadequate care during the dying process.

Lack of Information Resources for the Public on Palliative and End-of-Life Care

Faced with a diagnosis of cancer, people often respond by gathering information about the cause of their ailment, treatment options, and advances in medical research. Patients find information from any number of sources—health professionals, family, friends, religious leaders, printed materials, telephone hotlines, mail order, and increasingly, the World Wide Web. The materials available, however, emphasize curative treatment and living as a cancer survivor to the relative exclusion of information on palliative care and end-of-life issues. Kesselheim, in Chapter 4 of the full report, analyzes the state of information available for those with advanced cancer who are likely to die from their disease.

Physicians are often the first, and remain the most important, source of information for a large proportion of patients about all aspects of a cancer diagnosis and treatment.

Information Producers: National Cancer Institute, American Cancer Society, and Others

NCI and the American Cancer Society (ACS) write the majority of educational materials for cancer patients, in the form of booklets, pamphlets, and fact sheets, and make them freely available in a variety of ways. Most of the materials deal with cancer prevention, descriptions of various cancers and their treatments, clinical trials, and survivorship concerns. Only recently have NCI and ACS begun publishing materials related to end-of-life issues.

NCI produces one publication, *Advanced Cancer: Living Each Day* (1998), aimed at dying patients and booklets for some specific end-of-life concerns: *Eating Hints for Cancer Patients* (1998), *Get Relief from Cancer Pain* (1994), and *Pain Control* (2000, published in conjunction with ACS). NCI's Physician Data Query (PDQ) has a section dealing with "Supportive Care Topics," covering the major symptoms at the end of life. There are also "Cancer Facts," information sheets about hospice care and national and local cancer support organizations.

Finally, NCI's Cancer Information Service (CIS) comprises 19 resource centers across the country that answer calls to "1-800-4-CANCER." CIS representatives mail patients NCI-produced and other approved materials, according to the type and stage of cancer and the caller's requests.

In addition to distributing NCI material, ACS offers its own booklets, including one directed at end-of-life care, called *Caring for the Patient with Cancer at Home* (1998).

Overall, the easily available information about palliative and end-of-life care is inadequate. The few publications mentioned are among hundreds of cancer-related publications that ignore the dimension of advanced disease and death from cancer. For instance, the NCI booklet *What You Need to Know About Ovarian Cancer* (1993) mentions nothing about the possibility that a patient might die of an ovarian tumor, despite the fact that this cancer often is diagnosed in late stages, with little hope for long-term survival. While the ACS document on lung cancer relays the generally low overall survival rates and suggests "supportive care" as a viable choice for patients diagnosed as Stage IV non-small cell lung cancer, these paragraphs are given less space than highly investigational treatments such as immunotherapy and gene therapy. The materials that NCI and ACS offer to deal with other end-of-life symptoms (e.g., pain, loss of appetite) also mention little about death and dying. A factor limiting the effective reach of even the few relevant NCI and ACS materials that exist is that most are currently available only in English.

Many other organizations issue educational materials and distribute NCI and ACS booklets, and a few organizations dedicate themselves specifically to end-of-life concerns in cancer care. In general, these organizations have low visibility, and even if they have good information, most patients will never hear about them. In addition, the organizations themselves have limited abilities to adapt information to the individual needs of patients. Most patients who call, no matter how advanced their condition is, receive the same introductory packet and pamphlets, which are likely to have little relevance for patients with advanced, recurrent, or terminal cancer.

Pharmaceutical companies have begun producing information about symptom control that, not surprisingly, concentrates on their own products. A pharmaceutical firm that produces an antiemetic has little reason to alert people to competing products or approaches, much less treatments for other symptoms.

End-of-Life Information from Health Care Providers

Physicians remain the primary source of information for patients about end-of-life care, but patients are often reluctant to bring up the topics of death and dying, so physicians themselves must initiate discussions if they are to take place (Pfeifer et al., 1994). Many physicians are not well prepared for this task, however, either by training or by experience. They may avoid it altogether, or if they attempt to inform and counsel patients, they may be unaware that the patient (and family members) may not fully understand the information or may be overwhelmed by too much information. Physicians and other health care providers, even at major cancer centers, may not have access to information resources that would facilitate informing their patients.

Another illustration relates to advance directives, mandated by law in some states and by hospital policy in some institutions. Many physicians and nurses will admit that these forms are often handed to newly admitted patients, among a large stack of paperwork, with little explanation.

Finally, even though many NCI-designated cancer centers might advertise themselves as extremely effective sources of patient education and information, the number of people who have access to these institutions is limited, both geographically and because most patients simply are not treated in cancer centers. Most of the centers are currently reluctant (or unable) to provide information to outsiders who are not patients at their institution.

Current deficiencies in communication between patients and their physicians about end-of-life issues have many other origins. Poor provider communication skills and knowledge of end-of-life issues, and a health care market that discourages referrals to hospice and rewards medical procedures and treatments over cognitive therapy, also can contribute to poor communication by health care providers.

End-of-Life Information from the World Wide Web

The Internet has emerged as a powerful influence in all information-gathering activities, and cancer and end-of-life information is no exception. The interactive nature of the World Wide Web allows people not only to access static sites, but also to communicate with counselors or support groups and watch or listen to audiovisual clips.

Nearly all of the cancer organizations that patients and their family members have traditionally contacted by phone or letter have now constructed Web pages to disseminate their resources. Exclusively Web-based sources of patient education and information have also emerged. A search for "end-of-life issues" leads to reviews of palliative care handbooks, hospice information sites, video downloads, and numerous articles and hyperlinks. NCI lists a number of links on its Web site, including major organizations and Web sites devoted to hospice.

The biggest hurdle to effective use of the Web is access. Surfing the Internet requires a computer, a modem, and a Web browser, as well as facility in navigating. A larger problem, in the long run, is the variable quality of information on the Internet, the accuracy of which is unregulated.

Lack of Reliable Data on Quality of Life and Quality of Care at the End of Life

There is sufficient information from recent studies to demonstrate that cancer patients are consistently undertreated for pain, are underdiagnosed for their psychological distress, and have significant economic barriers to getting palliative care and that health care professionals identify their lack of both knowledge and training, as well as ability to obtain effective services for their patients, as major barriers to providing adequate care. At the same time, we have little understanding of the particular dying experiences of most patients with cancer—where they die, who cares for them as they are dying, what the quality of such care is, whether guidelines are in fact being followed, and whether these things are changing over time. This lack of information hampers our ability to develop a clear policy agenda and will, in the future, impede monitoring trends to determine whether interventions are having their intended effects.

Knowing how well we're doing or whether things are getting better in end-of-life care requires some routinely collected information, as well as specific studies. New data collection efforts might be necessary, but it may be possible to make better use of data already being collected, including those collected for other purposes. HCFA's claims for Medicare reimbursement constitute a major resource on their own, and because it is becoming increasingly feasible to link these "claims data" to those from other systems and surveys, they may prove an even more powerful data source.

The needs for an in-depth assessment of the information potential of current data sources and for an assessment of future needs are identified in this report but are not within the scope of work. The NCPB plans a comprehensive follow-on report to delve into this topic and will defer recommendations related to data collection until that report is complete.

Low Level of Public Investment in Palliative and End-of-Life Care Research

Despite billions of dollars spent on research in cancer biology and cancer therapeutics, there has been little investment in research that might significantly alleviate the physical and psychological distress of patients at the end of life. In Part II of the full report, Cleeland (Chapter 8) reports that compared to the rest of the cancer research establishment, research directed at cancer-related symptom management is poorly organized, poorly conceptualized, underfunded, and dependent on an insufficient number of well-trained researchers.

The feasibility of symptom control research has been demonstrated. Studies of the epidemiology of symptoms, behavioral research, health services research, and basic research, as well as clinical trials, have already produced benefits that have been translated into better care. Although the amount of improvement has not been well studied, it is very possible that patients now experience less distress related to medical procedures, that pain is somewhat better managed, and that there is wider recognition of and attention to end-of-life issues such as patient preference for end-of-life decisionmaking. Research has also documented the gaps between current care and optimal care and has identified very specific obstacles that could be addressed to improve care.

Perhaps less obvious has been a maturation of research methods that should facilitate rapid progress of research in this area. Subjective reports of patients about quality of life and symptoms are increasingly accepted as reasonable measures for clinical and laboratory research. Quality-of-life outcomes—including aspects of symptom control—have become more accepted as clinical trial end points. New technologies offer unique opportunities to understand the nature, mechanisms, and expression of symptoms that were not possible a few years ago (e.g., new brain imaging techniques to study pain and depression) and, further, to see how treatment affects them. Developments in neurobiology have opened windows to a better understanding of end-of-life symptoms. Exciting new agents that could provide better control of most of the symptoms of the dying process have been and are being developed. There is a real possibility that individual variation in symptom expression may be better understood through progress in genetic science. It can no longer be said that tools to advance the area are lacking, and there is also no lack of research targets.

The understanding of pain, although more advanced than that of other symptoms, still has enormous gaps to be filled. This finding is confirmed and detailed in a January 2001 AHRQ Evidence Report/Technology Assessment, *Management of Cancer Pain* (AHRQ, 2001), which concludes:

> Randomized controlled trials establish that many current treatment modalities can individually reduce cancer pain. These trials constitute 1 percent of the published literature on cancer pain, enroll one in 10,000 patients at risk for cancer pain in industrialized countries, are often heterogeneous, and use poor methodology. Leading investigators in the area of cancer pain relief have repeatedly called for improving the quality of trials in this area. The quantity and quality of scientific evidence on cancer pain relief still, however, compare unfavorably with the great deal that is known about other high-impact conditions, including cancer

itself. In the current era of patient-centered care, closing this gap should be a high research priority.

Our understanding of symptoms other than pain is much more primitive. Research examining ways of improving the care given to patients with advanced cancer is just beginning. Methods for studying and providing for the more complex subjective needs of patients (spiritual, existential) have to be developed. Few of the common practices of caring for patients with advanced cancer have been subjected to careful randomized clinical trials, impeding the provision of evidence-based practice recommendations.

Cleeland has laid out a research agenda for the most important symptoms in the disciplines of basic science, epidemiology, social-behavioral research, health services research, and clinical trials. Specific opportunities and currently unmet research needs in symptom control are outlined in Table 3.

END-OF-LIFE AND PALLIATIVE CARE: EVOLUTION OF THE ISSUE

Until the early part of the twentieth century, most Americans died of infectious diseases, many in childhood and middle age. Then, virtually every serious illness, including cancer, spelled a fairly rapid course to death. Those who survived to old age and developed the chronic diseases that the majority of people now die from had shorter trajectories until death, with few experiencing prolonged periods of critical illness leading up to death. Malignancies were identified only when large or in a critical location, and most often, no treatments were available that substantially altered the course. The fact that cancer patients often lingered a few months, often with disturbing appearance, odors, and suffering, undoubtedly contributed to cancer's special position of abhorrence in the popular mythology. Now, patients with cancer often live much longer because of better prevention, earlier diagnosis, and treatments that prolong survival, resulting in longer periods of adaptation to cancer as a chronic debilitating disease. However, most still eventually die from the cancer.

After World War II, the health care system grew rapidly, with hospitals assuming a place of prominence. The emphasis was on acute care, which led to what has been referred to as the "medicalization" of death, confining it largely to hospitals. By the late 1960s and early 1970s, a grassroots movement had taken hold in the United States that began focusing on the development of volunteer hospice programs, in an attempt to "demedicalize" death. This reached its peak in 1982, when the Medicare hospice benefit was developed. From 1982 to the present, hospice has become more and more available under Medicare (although with the prob-

TABLE 3 Symptom Control Research Opportunities and Unmet Needs

Symptom	Basic	Clinical or Health Services
Pain	• Elucidate basic mechanisms of visceral and neuropathic pain; identify new treatments • Identify modifications of nervous system involved in chronic pain perception • Find new compounds with more precise analgesic action and fewer side effects • Find molecular basis of pain signaling, receptor modification due to pain, and ways to modify • Identify forebrain structures that modulate responses to "painful" signals • Determine receptor affinities of different opioids	• Determine why so many patients have poorly controlled pain • Study ways to improve cancer pain management • Determine effectiveness of treatments for neuropathic pain • Determine effects of cancer on tolerance to opioid analgesics and how pain can be managed in already tolerant patients • Determine side-effect profiles of different opioids • Conduct trials of intrathecal delivery of novel analgesics
Anorexia or Cachexia	• Elucidate roles for various cytokines in cachexia • Elucidate roles of food regulatory peptides in cachexia	Conduct clinical trials of • Proinflammatory mediators • Appetite stimulants • Anticatabolic agents (e.g., neuropeptide agonists or antagonists, $beta_2$-adrenoceptor agonists) • Polyunsaturated fatty acids, n-3 fatty acids, fish oil • Anabolic agents (especially hormonal) • Anticytokines (e.g., megestrol acetate, medroxyprogesterone acetate, thalidomide, melatonin)

Cognitive failure: delirium, temporary and permanent cognitive impairment	• Elucidate underlying mechanisms of delirium and cognitive impairment
	• Identify role of cancer disease process in cognitive impairment
	• Determine how biological therapies (e.g., interferon alpha, interleukin-2) produce cognitive impairment
	• Find biological markers for patients most at risk of
		• Develop standardized assessment for delirium
		• Determine prevalence, nature, and current treatments for delirium and cognitive impairment
		• Conduct clinical trials of
		  – Drugs used empirically for delirium (haloperidol) and cognitive impairment (methylphenidate)
		  – stimulants for cognitive

TABLE 3 Continued

Symptom	Basic	Clinical or Health Services
	delirium or cognitive impairment	impairment • Require neuropsychological assessments in cancer treatment trials to determine whether drugs are causing cognitive impairment
Dyspnea	• Standardize measurement and assessment • Develop animal model • Determine relationship of dyspnea to anemia in chronic illness • Determine role of respiratory muscle metabolism and function • Elucidate link between cachexia, tumor necrosis factor, muscle fatigue or weakness, and dyspnea	• Study prevalence, severity, and current treatment • Conduct clinical trials of opioids by different routes of administration • Conduct clinical trials of other agents (e.g., corticosteroids)
Fatigue	• Explore new agents (e.g., anticytokines) • Develop animal models • Explore common pathways for fatigue and other symptoms	Conduct clinical trials of • Stimulant therapies • Current anticytokines • Selective serotonin receptor uptake inhibitors (SSRIs) • Exercise • Behavioral interventions
Gastrointestinal symptoms	• Study relationship of terminal nausea to other symptoms of advanced disease • Determine mechanisms of terminal and treatment-induced nausea	• Study prevalence, severity and current treatment of terminal nausea • Conduct clinical trials of agents for nausea of advanced disease and for bowel obstruction
Psychiatric or affective symptoms	• Develop animal model for cancer-related affective disturbances • Study mechanisms of depression unique to cancer and its treatment	• Describe current management in advanced disease • Conduct clinical trials of standard antidepressants, especially SSRIs; stimulant therapies (e.g., methylphenidate); and agents for terminal agitation or restlessness • Consider trials of novel agents: "empathogens"

SOURCE: Cleeland, Chapter 8 of the full report.

lems alluded to earlier). Over the period 1994 through 1998, 45 percent of all beneficiaries who died from cancer used some hospice services, and for 1998 alone, more than half of all cancer patients who died used hospice services. Although use by people dying from other conditions has grown considerably, far fewer use hospice (e.g., 10 percent of beneficiaries dying of congestive heart failure from 1994 through 1998 used hospice, as did 20 percent of those dying of Alzheimer's and other dementias) (Hogan et al., 2000).

Even thoroughly tested, effective measures to improve the quality of life of dying patients through symptom control have not been widely adopted; in contrast, the most marginal improvements in chemotherapy to extend life—often at reduced quality—diffuse remarkably quickly. Our desire to evade and avoid the events associated with death pervades society. It could be argued that no institution mirrors society as well as the U.S. Congress. In their recommendations for funding the National Cancer Institute—approaching $4 billion for fiscal year 2001—the House of Representatives and the Senate Appropriations Committees both detail a rich research agenda that covers many specific types of cancer, screening and early detection, and finding cures, but not a single word about research to help alleviate the symptoms of cancer, either for those who survive or for those who die.

Societal attitudes have evolved, to some extent, as a result of public airing of the issues. Discussions about dying have become more acceptable, and patients and families have increasingly played greater roles in deciding on the goals and details of treatment. Yet the task of ensuring that the best care is available when people are dying and that avoidable distress is minimized to provide the best "quality of death" has to be accomplished even in the face of reluctance of the dying and those around them to grapple with key issues and necessary decisions. Fortunately, there is progress to report.

A constellation of factors has put palliative care on the agenda as a medical issue: the development of technology-intensive approaches for patients with advanced disease, advances in treatment for cancer patients and patients with AIDS, a large and aging elderly population, a growing population of patients with significant neurological and neurodegenerative diseases requiring continuous care, and limitations in health care resources. All of these issues have come together at a time when the country is trying to address how it cares for patients with serious life-threatening illness and the controversies of withholding and withdrawing care, physician-assisted suicide, euthanasia, and a U.S. Supreme Court decision on physician-assisted suicide that asserts a right to palliative care. It is also a time of medical advance and the potential for much greater advances.

The lead in tackling palliative care and improved end-of-life care has been taken largely by private foundations, in particular, the Robert Wood

Johnson Foundation, the Nathan Cummings Foundation, the Fetzer Institute, the Commonwealth Fund, and the Project on Death in America, which together have underwritten a wide range of innovative research, training, and public awareness programs. They have laid the groundwork for moving forward, but the foundation focus does not represent a permanent presence in the field and is likely to be scaled back in the future.

Federal government efforts took shape in hospitals run by the Department of Veterans Affairs (VA), in their role as caregivers for elderly and dying veterans. VA developed a faculty scholars program in palliative care, the requirement that pain be recorded as a "fifth vital sign" for all patients, and hospice programs at all its major hospitals. Other early government steps include the Medicare hospice benefit and the efforts of the Health Resources and Services Administration (HRSA) in care provided within the prison system, as well as for patients with AIDS.

THE 1990s: SIGNAL EFFORTS AND EVENTS AROUND PALLIATIVE AND END-OF-LIFE CARE

Central among the early prime movers in palliative care has been the Robert Wood Johnson Foundation (RWJF), which funded the groundbreaking Study to Understand Prognoses and Preferences for Outcomes and Risks of Treatment. RWJF has continued to shine the spotlight on end-of-life needs through its "Last Acts" program, which encourages activities at local levels and other activities; its "Promoting Excellence in End-of-Life Care" program (see Box 2); and others, including sponsorship of a recent six-hour public television special on palliative and end-of-life care ("On Our Own Terms: Moyers on Dying," September 2000).

Some of the touchstone events in end-of-life and palliative care are described in the sections that follow.

The Study to Understand Prognoses and Preferences for Outcomes and Risks of Treatment

Asked to name the most influential phenomenon in moving end-of-life care in the 1990s, most who know the field would probably name SUPPORT—the Study to Understand Prognoses and Preferences for Outcomes and Risks of Treatment. SUPPORT was a two-stage research project, beginning with an observational study of aspects of end-of-life care, followed by a randomized intervention trial to try to improve the quality of care found in the first stage, with the emphasis on communication between caregivers and patients. A companion study, HELP—the Hospitalized Elderly Longitudinal Project—was similar to the first stage of SUPPORT, but included only the very old, people 80 years and over (see Box 2 for a

---

Box 2
SUPPORT

Although the Study to Understand Prognoses and Preferences for Outcomes and Risks of Treatment—SUPPORT—came to public attention in the 1990s, it was conceived in the early 1980s, at a time when costs for high-technology medical interventions were increasing rapidly and people had begun to question the appropriateness of using all available measures to extend briefly the lives of people with untreatable, soon fatal, conditions. The Robert Wood Johnson Foundation, sole sponsor of SUPPORT and HELP, held a meeting in 1985 to discuss this. Subsequently, it asked Drs. William Knaus and Joanne Lynn to propose a study to improve the care of critically ill, hospitalized adults, specifically through improving the match between what patients wanted and the care they actually received.

A two-stage process was planned: Phase I was observational, and Phase II was a randomized trial testing an intervention tailored to address problems identified in Phase I. Planning, pilot testing, and recruitment took several years. Defining which patients would be eligible for the study was pivotal. The investigators chose conditions that were common and often fatal; that required important decisions during hospitalization; and that had stable treatment possibilities, to ensure that prognostic estimates would be similar throughout the study (this is one reason HIV/AIDS was not selected). Patients' conditions had to be severe enough that about half would die within six months. The conditions selected were

- acute respiratory failure,
- chronic obstructive pulmonary disease,
- congestive heart failure,
- coma,
- cirrhosis,
- advanced colon or non-small cell lung cancer, and
- multiorgan system failure with sepsis or malignancy.

Between 1989 and 1991, a full complement of 4,301 patients had been recruited to Phase I at the five large hospitals around the country that had been selected (out of 55 applications) as study sites. The following are key Phase I findings:

- Patients with advanced life-threatening illnesses could be interviewed successfully about their treatment preferences.
- Physicians often misunderstood patient preferences, especially when patients did not want high-technology, life-extending care.
- Do-not-resuscitate (DNR) orders were often written very late—just before

---

description of the studies). SUPPORT and HELP were funded solely by the Robert Wood Johnson Foundation at more than $29 million, the largest project ever funded by RWJF (Phillips et al., 2000).

The SUPPORT randomized trial is "negative," in that the interventions did not improve quality of care in the hoped-for ways. The irony is that SUPPORT and HELP focused the attention of professionals and the public death—and many patients died after long stays in intensive care units (ICUs) either comatose or with mechanical ventilation.

- Survival time could be better predicted by a computerized model with appropriate data inputs than by an individual physician.
- An unexpectedly large percentage of patients experienced substantial pain across all diagnoses.
- The study participants were younger than anticipated (median age less than 65), which led to HELP, a companion study of patients more than 80 years of age.

The Phase II intervention employed a skilled nurse specialist to interact with patients and their families, staff, and the intervention physicians. Specifically,

- physicians were given detailed prognostic information for each patient on survival, outcome if cardiopulmonary resuscitation was used, and prospect of severe disability;
- nurse specialists talked to patients and families about their specific wishes regarding treatment and communicated that information to the physicians and nurses treating the patient; and
- physicians were given written information regarding each patient's wishes about treatment, including pain control and the use of technology-intensive measures (e.g., CPR).

All participating physicians also were given feedback on the overall results of the observational phase of the study, characterizing the shortcomings of physician-patient communication, pain, and the timing of DNR orders.

A form of "cluster randomization" (by physician specialty and study site) was used to assign patients to either the intervention or the usual-care groups (see SUPPORT Principal Investigators, 1995, for details). The evidence after enrollment of 4,804 patients in two years was examined for five outcomes:

1. median time until the DNR order was written,
2. agreement between patient and physician regarding the DNR order,
3. number of days spent in an "undesirable state" (e.g., comatose, on mechanical ventilation, in ICUs),
4. percentage of patients in substantial pain, and
5. median resource use (in 1993 dollars).

None of the outcomes was better for patients in the intervention group than for those in the control group.

on care of the dying—stories about the project made front-page news in the national press—in a way that nothing else had. SUPPORT also catalyzed new thinking about the nature of the problems underlying care at the end of life and about what changes would be needed to fix them. Simplistically, we moved from hoping that doing A, B, and C to improve communication would result in better care (widely believed by experts to be the answer before SUPPORT), to an understanding that much broader system-wide and society-wide changes would have to take place. The depth and richness of the studies, beyond this single finding, are hinted at by the 100 or so journal articles that have probed SUPPORT data (Phillips et al., 2000).

The failure of the planned interventions spurred the interested community to try to understand what went wrong and what could be done differently. This led RWJF to begin its Last Acts campaign, an effort to improve end-of-life care at the grassroots level that now has more than 400 members (Schroeder, 1999), and funding of demonstration programs to reduce the identified barriers to high-quality care for those who are dying.

Other Key Foundation Commitments

The Project on Death in America (PDIA) (www.soros.org/death) has committed $30 million to improving end-of-life care through its Faculty Scholars Program, grant programs, and special initiatives. The 70 or so faculty scholars that have been funded by PDIA serve as role models and clinical researchers in academic medical centers around the United States (and a few in Canada). About one-third of them are oncologists involved in direct patient care and directing palliative care programs.

The Nathan Cummings Foundation, together with the Commonwealth Fund, supported a major study of nearly 1,000 dying patients (most with cancer, heart disease, or chronic lung disease) and their caregivers. This is one of eight major research projects designed to expand the nation's understanding of the dying experience and find ways to improve it.

The Milbank Foundation (www.milbank.org) sponsored the development and publication of *Principles for Care of Patients at the End of Life: An Emerging Consensus Among the Specialties of Medicine* (Cassel and Foley, 1999), a document now signed onto by at least 17 health professional societies that have agreed to incorporate its principles into their professional education activities and residency training programs.

The Institute of Medicine

Another milestone was the 1997 report *Approaching Death: Improving Care at the End of Life* from the Institute of Medicine (1997). This was the first major national report covering the range of end-of-life issues, with evidence-based recommendations (see Box 3). It received widespread national attention and continues to be cited as a reference and source of guidance for improving end-of-life care. This report builds on the earlier report and its recommendations. (The reader is referred to the 1997 report for a thorough review of issues up to that time.) The 1999 National Cancer

---

Box 3
RECOMMENDATIONS AND FUTURE DIRECTIONS—
From *Approaching Death: Improving Care at the End of Life*
(IOM, 1997)

Seven recommendations address different decisionmakers and different deficiencies in care at the end of life. Each applies generally to people approaching death including those for whom death is imminent and those with serious, eventually fatal illnesses who may live for some time. Each is intended to contribute to the achievement of a compassionate care system that dying people and those close to them can rely on for respectful and effective care.

Recommendation 1: People with advanced, potentially fatal illnesses and those close to them should be able to expect and receive reliable, skillful, and supportive care.

Recommendation 2: Physicians, nurses, social workers, and other health professionals must commit themselves to improving care for dying patients and to using existing knowledge effectively to prevent and relieve pain and other symptoms.

Recommendation 3: Because many problems in care stem from system problems, policymakers, consumer groups, and purchasers of health care should work with health care practitioners, organizations, and researchers to:

a) strengthen methods for measuring the quality of life and other outcomes of care for dying patients and those close to them;
b) develop better tools and strategies for improving the quality of care and holding health care organizations accountable for care at the end of life;
c) revise mechanisms for financing care so that they encourage rather than impede good end-of-life care and sustain rather than frustrate coordinated systems of excellent care; and
d) reform drug prescription laws, burdensome regulations, and state medical board policies and practices that impede effective use of opioids to relieve pain and suffering.

Recommendation 4: Educators and other health professionals should initiate changes in undergraduate, graduate, and continuing education to ensure that practitioners have relevant attitudes, knowledge, and skills to care well for dying patients.

Recommendation 5: Palliative care should become, if not a medical specialty, at least a defined area of expertise, education, and research.

Recommendation 6: The nation's research establishment should define and implement priorities for strengthening the knowledge base for end-of-life care.

Recommendation 7: A continuing public discussion is essential to develop a better understanding of the modern experience of dying, the options available to patients and families, and the obligations of communities to those approaching death.

Policy Board report *Ensuring Quality Cancer Care* (IOM, 1999) has already been mentioned.

The President's Cancer Panel

The 1997-1998 report of the President's Cancer Panel[1] (PCP) was entitled *Cancer Care Issues in the United States: Quality of Care, Quality of Life*, with a major focus on the need for NCI to fund research and training across the spectrum of care, including cancer prevention, cancer control, rehabilitation, palliation, and end-of-life care (President's Cancer Panel, 1998). The report states:

> The quality of care provided to dying patients remains woefully inadequate and is a major failure of our health care system. Dying patients frequently face abandonment by their physicians and inadequate pain and other symptom control when treatment with curative intent is no longer tenable.

The PCP developed its report after a series of meetings around the country, at which a wide range of individuals—from the medical treatment and research communities, industry, the advocacy community, and the public at large—presented testimony about the quality of cancer care in the United States. Those who spoke about palliative and end-of-life care reinforced earlier findings (PCP, 1998):

> Speakers emphasized the need for a compassionate and humane system of care for cancer patients at the end of life, including improved financing of hospice care, expanding the availability of palliative care approaches from hospice programs to cancer centers (including offering palliative care as an option in all clinical trials), establishing a focal point for palliative care research at the NCI, improving health care professional education about palliative care, and fostering more honest health professional and public dialogue about dying. A number of respected organizations, including the American Society of Clinical Oncology, the Institute of Medicine, and the World Health Organization, have developed reports and accompanying recommendations to address the deeply ingrained obstacles to compassionate end of life care for people with cancer. However, implementation of these recommendations and their integration into the standard of care is slow.

---

[1]The President's Cancer Panel, consisting of three individuals, was created by congressional charter in 1971 to "monitor the development and execution of the activities of the National Cancer Program, and ... report directly to the President."

Among the panel's recommendations, the following relate to training and research in end-of-life and palliative care:

Training is needed to improve the ability of physicians and other health professionals to . . .:

Acknowledge that death and end of life issues are a part of the cancer experience for some patients, and provide more comprehensive and compassionate care to dying patients and their families.

The panel also stated:

Continued funding across the research spectrum is needed to continue the flow of discovery that leads to improvements in care across the cancer continuum. Research efforts should focus particularly on improving interventions in the areas of cancer prevention, cancer control, rehabilitation, palliation, and end of life care, and on outcomes research. In addition, targeted funding may be needed for behavioral and other research to improve quality of care in vulnerable populations, including those with low income and/or educational levels, differing cultures, the elderly, and rural populations.

Medicare Payment Advisory Commission (MedPAC)

MedPAC is an independent federal organization that was established by Congress for advice on issues affecting the Medicare program. Chapters devoted to end-of-life care appeared in recent major reports (MedPAC, 1998, 1999) including, in 1999, recommendations for the Medicare program and the Department of Health and Human Services, more broadly. They directed the Secretary of Health and Human Services to

• make end-of-life care a national quality improvement priority for Medicare+Choice and traditional Medicare;
• support research on care at the end of life and work with nongovernmental organizations as they (1) educate the health care profession and the public about care at the end of life and (2) develop measures to accredit health care organizations and provide public accountability for the quality of end-of-life care;
• sponsor projects to develop and test measures of the quality of end-of-life care for Medicare beneficiaries, and enlist quality improvement organizations and Medicare+Choice plans to implement quality improvement programs for care at the end of life; and
• promote advance care planning by practitioners and patients well before terminal health crises occur.

As yet, neither the Congress nor the Secretary has responded to these MedPAC recommendations.

Other Organizations and Efforts

A variety of professional and trade organizations, consumer groups, pharmaceutical companies, and others have taken positive steps related to palliative and end-of-life care, only the most prominent of which are touched on here. The American Society of Clinical Oncology (ASCO) is the main professional organization for practicing oncologists. In 1998, it took two important steps. First, ASCO published a position statement on cancer care during the last phase of life (ASCO, 1998), outlining the role of the oncologist, identifying impediments to achieving the best care, and recommending solutions. The details of the position statement flow from the belief that "it is the oncologists' responsibility to care for their patients in a continuum that extends from the moment of diagnosis throughout the course of the illness." The statement goes on, "In addition to appropriate anticancer treatment, this includes symptom control and psychosocial support during all phases of care, including those during the last phase of life."

Also in 1998, ASCO surveyed its membership in the first nationwide inquiry into end-of-life practices. The survey asked about education and training, current practice, perceived barriers to the delivery of care, decisionmaking vignettes about the management of patients, and individual experiences with terminal patients. The results, which have been presented at meetings and have begun to appear in print, confirm many of the deficiencies that have been recognized in caring for dying patients, but coming from the oncology community, they have hit with added force (see Box 4 for key survey findings).

For the long term, ASCO has placed high priority on developing its program called "Optimizing Cancer Care: The Importance of Symptom Management." The curriculum consists of 32 modules covering specific symptoms and symptom control issues (e.g., ascites, breaking bad news, depression, lymphedema). Modules are designed to get information into manageable pieces for practicing oncologists in a way that is concise and information-dense. The program has been featured at national ASCO meetings and will be featured at all yearly state ASCO meetings. ASCO plans to make it available on CD-ROM, on-line, and in print.

The Joint Commission on the Accreditation of Healthcare Organizations is the first national accrediting body to develop mandatory standards for pain assessment and management. JCAHO, which accredits the majority of hospitals and other health care organizations (including hospices), will begin evaluating the hospitals, home care agencies, nursing homes, behavioral health facilities, outpatient clinics, and health plans it inspects for compliance with the new standards in 2001. The organizations will be required to

- recognize the right of patients to appropriate assessment and management of pain;
- assess the existence and, if so, the nature and intensity of pain in all patients;
- record the results of the assessment in a way that facilitates regular reassessment and follow-up;
- determine and ensure staff competency in pain assessment and management, and address pain assessment and management in the orientation of all new staff;
- establish policies and procedures that support the appropriate prescription or ordering of effective pain medications;
- educate patients and their families about effective pain management; and
- address patient needs for symptom management in the discharge planning process.

The standards were developed collaboratively with the University of Wisconsin-Madison Medical School, as part of a project funded by RWJF to make pain assessment and management a priority in the nation's health care system (JCAHO Web site, http://www.jcaho.org/news/nb207.html).

CURRENT NIH INVOLVEMENT IN PALLIATIVE AND END-OF-LIFE CARE

The National Institutes of Health responded to recommendations in the IOM (1997) report and to the widely publicized SUPPORT findings with an initiative in symptom control and palliative care at a meeting in November 2000. This was by no means NIH's first recognition of research needs in palliative care. A prominent earlier effort was a 1979 interdisciplinary meeting on pain, which provided some of the stimulus for advances in pain control in the 1980s and 1990s, and a follow-up meeting in the early 1990s. Despite these activities, no standing program was ever developed.

The main event of the 1997 effort was a workshop that was cosponsored by the National Institute of Nursing Research (NINR), the Division of AIDS Research of the National Institute of Allergy and Infectious Diseases (NIAID), NCI, and the Office of Alternative Medicine to target research needs in palliative care. The research workshop "Symptoms in Terminal Illness" had three principal goals:

Box 4
THE ASCO SURVEY

In 1998, American Society of Clinical Oncology conducted the first and only large-scale survey of U.S. oncologists about their experiences in providing care to dying patients. The questionnaire consisted of 118 questions about end-of-life care under eight headings (Hilden et al., 2001):

1. education and training,
2. current practice,
3. perceived barriers to the delivery of care,
4. decisionmaking,
5. vignettes about the management of patients,
6. individual experiences with terminal patients,
7. the role of ASCO in improving care, and
8. demographics and practice characteristics of the respondents.

All U.S. oncologists who reported that they managed patients at the end of life, and were ASCO members, were eligible for the survey, a total of 6,645 (the small number of ASCO members from England and Canada was also included). About 40 percent (2,645) responded (see table below) (Emanuel, 2000). No information is available to compare the characteristics of those who responded with those who did not.

This survey documented serious shortcomings in the training and current practices of a large proportion of oncologists. Among the key findings are the following:

• Most oncologists have not had adequate formal training in the key skills needed for them to provide excellent palliative and end-of-life care. Less than one-third reported their formal training "very helpful" in communicating with dying patients, coordinating their care, shifting to palliative care, or beginning hospice care. About 40 percent found their training very helpful in managing dying patients' symptoms.

• Slightly more than half (56 percent) reported "trial and error in clinical practice" as one important source of learning about end-of-life care. About 45 percent also ranked role models during fellowships and in practice as important. Traumatic patient experiences ranked higher as a source of learning than did lectures during fellowship, medical school role models, and clinical clerkships.

• Only 25 percent reported end-of-life care as highly satisfying; about 40 percent thought it intellectually satisfying; and 63 percent, emotionally satisfying. Substantial numbers reported a sense of failure when a patient becomes terminally ill (10 percent), and a similar proportion reported anxiety and strong emotions when faced with follow-up meetings with dying patients and managing difficult symptoms. About twice as many reported anxiety and strong emotions when they had to tell a patient that his or her condition would lead to death.

• The large majority of oncologists report that they are highly competent in managing patients' cancer-related end-of-life symptoms, including pain (95 percent report high competency), constipation (91 percent), nausea and vomiting (93 percent), fever, and neutropenia (89 percent); somewhat fewer report high competency in managing shortness of breath (79 percent), anorexia (63 percent), and depression (57 percent).

• Very few oncologists (6 percent) feel they can arrange for their patients to get all the services they need. About half report getting their patients "almost all" of what they need, but the rest report that their patients get less. More than half (56 percent) report that a palliative care team is either not available or not easy to access. Smaller but still substantial proportions report lack of availability or difficult access to hospital-based hospice (28 percent), a pain service (18 percent), outpatient case management (17 percent), and psychosocial support services (15 percent).

• The barriers to providing adequate end-of-life care most often cited are patient and family denial that death is approaching and unrealistic expectations for curative treatment. Other factors (e.g., laws restricting opioid usage) are reported as frequent problems by only 6 percent.

• Reimbursement practices are reported as frequent barriers to providing good care. Slightly more than one-quarter report insufficient reimbursement for time spent in discussion with patients and families as the "most troublesome" among reimbursement barriers. A much larger group (41 percent) reports lack of coverage for unskilled home health services as the most troublesome aspect. Also troublesome are restrictive referral networks and lack of appropriate coding categories (diagnosis-related groups) for end-of-life and palliative care.

• In answer to questions about a series of patient vignettes, respondents indicated what course of treatment they favored. As an example, for a patient with locally advanced lung cancer who "failed first line chemotherapy," 3 percent would recommend hospice and the rest would recommend additional chemotherapy (paclitaxel or a phase I trial); after failing paclitaxel, 19 percent would refer to hospice and the rest to additional chemotherapy; failing the third-line treatment, 80 percent would refer the patient to hospice care, but the remaining 20 percent would consider additional chemotherapy.

Attitudes and practices relating to euthanasia and "physician-assisted suicide" were elicited in various questions, with the following points emerging (Emanuel et al., 2000a):

• About one-third of the respondents had been asked to perform either euthanasia or "physician-assisted suicide" within the previous year, and nearly two-thirds had had such requests at some time during their career; 4 percent had performed one or both within the previous year, and 13 percent, at some time in their career. Most instances were physician-assisted suicide (11 percent of respondents) rather than euthanasia (4 percent).

• Concern among oncologists about performing euthanasia and physician-assisted suicide limits their willingness to prescribe adequate doses of opioids to control pain. Oncologists who do not support euthanasia or physician-assisted suicide are less willing than others to increase opioid dosages for severe pain.

• Better training in end-of-life care and the ability to obtain good palliative care for patients are associated with a lower likelihood of oncologists' performing euthanasia or physician-assisted suicide.

Response Rate Among Specialties

	Medical Oncologists	Surgical Oncologists	Radiation Oncologists	Pediatric Oncologists
Eligible	5010	499	703	371
Responders	2129	128	203	172
Response Rate, %	42.5	25.7	28.9	46.4

1. to summarize the current state of knowledge concerning the most common symptoms associated with terminal illness;

2. to identify important needs and opportunities for research that would be appropriate for NIH funding; and

3. to initiate a process for enhancing interdisciplinary collaboration and interagency collaboration in research in palliative care.

The workshop was organized into four topic sessions that focused on specific symptom areas: pain, dyspnea, cognitive disturbances, and cachexia and wasting. A research agenda was developed from the workshop report (http://www.nih.gov/ninr/end-of-life.htm), and in 1998, the collaborating institutes issued a program announcement "Management of Symptoms at the End of Life," with a call for proposals addressing the following objectives:

- managing the transition to palliative care;
- understanding and managing pain and other symptoms, such as nausea and depression in the context of end-stage illness;
- measuring outcomes (e.g., relief of symptoms);
- measuring of quality of life in end-stage illness;
- investigating changes in patient status that influence nutrition and hydration choices in terminal illness; and
- documenting costs incurred by patients and family caregivers during end-stage illness.

About two dozen small grants were issued as a result of this program, most funded by NINR, and three by NCI. NINR, which is designated the lead institute for end-of-life care, maintains it as an area of special research interest and has issued "program announcements" calling for proposals in end-of-life care every year since 1998 (NCI is a cosponsor of these announcements but has no up-front financial commitment to funding projects). In 1999, NINR-awarded grants related to end-of-life care totaled $2.3 million, and an addition $1.7 million went to cancer-related research projects with some end-of-life component (Hudgings, 2000). While nursing-related research is needed, the bulk of research needs extend far beyond nursing and are closely allied with cancer treatment, the bailiwick of NCI.

Within NCI, control of pain and other symptoms, psychosocial distress, and end-of-life issues has been associated administratively with cancer control or cancer prevention, which may be limiting the opportunities for broader research. The portfolio of palliative and end-of-life projects is currently within the Division of Cancer Prevention, where it has a very low profile among the many other issues more clearly related to cancer prevention. In fact, no direct mention of palliative or end-of-life care appears on the NCI Web site in association with any unit within the institute (although pain and other symptoms are mentioned in various places). Although a more natural fit, palliative care research has never been included as a specific topic in the Division of Cancer Treatment and Diagnosis (DCTD), which takes in preclinical and clinical drug development and testing. Althoug not specifically excluding drugs for symptom control, the language describing the Cancer Therapy Evaluation Program within DCTD refers to developing and evaluating "anticancer agents" (NCI Web site, October 2000), which would generally be understood as treatments aimed directly at the cancers themselves, not agents for palliative care.

NCI currently designates 37 centers as Comprehensive Cancer Centers (as of December 2000). The designation of "comprehensive" is awarded based on a strong and diverse research program, but current requirements do not include a program in palliative care research.

Researchers are not prohibited from applying to divisions other than the Division of Cancer Prevention for symptom control or end-of-life research (e.g., DCTD), but it appears that appropriate review mechanisms may be lacking, placing such researchers at a competitive disadvantage. For example, none of the established cooperative clinical trial groups has a specific mandate to conduct trials in symptom control, and there is no "coordinating center" for such trials, such as those that exist for other areas of treatment research.

NCI Funding for Palliative Care Research and Training

In this report, the Board recommends strongly that NCI step up its commitment to research toward improving end-of-life and palliative care— including symptom control, psychosocial issues, shared decisionmaking, and related topics. NCI has provided an accounting of its fiscal year 1999 extramural funding for all research with components related to palliative care or hospice, totaling $24.5 million (Colbert, 2000). (Most grants supported activities that were not focused exclusively on palliative care, so NCI has apportioned the dollar amounts attributed to this category as some percentage of the total grant.) Of that total, $18.3 million went to specific projects or programs (Appendix A, Table A-1), and $6.1 million represents fractions of institutional grants (Appendix A, Table A-2). Grants included in the list are those dealing with

- any and all aspects of cancer pain research, including mechanism, prevention, therapy, measurement tools, and so forth.;
- hospice, defined as research dealing with formally organized supportive care of terminally ill patients either at home or in an institution; and
- "other palliative care," including any supportive care (e.g., psycho-

logical counseling, relief of nausea, or other symptom management) that is not coded as pain or hospice.

In addition to the research grants, $1.7 million was spent in 1999 on training grants related to end-of-life or palliative care (Begg, 2000). Altogether, the 1999 NCI expenditure on palliative and hospice care was just over $26 million, or about 0.9 percent of the total 1999 budget of $2.9 billion.

Conclusions and Recommendations

People with cancer suffer from an array of symptoms at all stages of the disease (and its treatment), though these are most frequent and severe in advanced stages. Much of the suffering could be alleviated if currently available symptom control measures were used more widely. For symptoms not amenable to relief by current measures, new approaches could be developed and tested, if even modest resources were made available. Both the use of current interventions and the development of new ones are hindered by the barriers discussed earlier (and in Part II of the full report). The National Cancer Policy Board's recommendations are intended to break down or lower the barriers to excellent palliative care for people with cancer today and for those who will develop it in years to come. The recommendations describe a series of initiatives directed largely—though not exclusively—at the federal government, which should be playing a more powerful role than it has done.

The recommendations are not laid out in parallel to the barriers, as earlier in this report. They have been consolidated as "packages" for particular organizations and entities, and some address more than one barrier. Recommendation 1, in particular, which focuses on the role of NCI-designated cancer centers, contains elements that address all the barriers.

NCI-designated cancer centers should play a central role as agents of national policy in advancing palliative care research and clinical practice, with initiatives that address many of the barriers identified in this report.

Recommendation 1: NCI should designate certain cancer centers, as well as some community cancer centers, as centers of excellence in symptom control and palliative care for both adults and children. The centers will deliver the best available care, as well as carrying out research, training, and treatment aimed at developing portable model programs that can be adopted by other cancer centers and hospitals. Activities should include, but not be limited to, the following:

- *formal testing and evaluation of new and existing practice guidelines for palliative and end-of-life care;*
- *pilot testing "quality indicators" for assessing end-of-life care at the level of the patient and the institution;*
- *incorporating the best palliative care into NCI-sponsored clinical trials;*
- *innovating in the delivery of palliative and end-of-life care, including collaboration with local hospice organizations;*
- *disseminating information about how to improve end-of-life care to other cancer centers and hospitals through a variety of media;*
- *uncovering the determinants of disparities in access to care by minority populations that should be served by the center and developing specific programs and initiatives to increase access; these might include educational activities for health care providers and the community, setting up outreach programs, and so forth;*
- *providing clinical and research training fellowships in medical and surgical oncology in end-of-life care for adult and pediatric patients; and*
- *creating faculty development programs in oncology, nursing, and social work; and*
- *providing in-service training for local hospice staff in new palliative care techniques.*

Recommendation 2: NCI should add the requirement of research in palliative care and symptom control for recognition as a "Comprehensive Cancer Center."

Practices and policies that govern payment for palliative care (in both public and private sectors) hinder delivery of the most appropriate mix of services for patients who could benefit from palliative care during the course of their illness and treatments.

Recommendation 3: The Health Care Financing Administration (HCFA) should fund demonstration projects for service delivery and reimbursement that integrate palliative care and potentially life-prolonging treatments throughout the course of disease.

Recommendation 4: Private insurers should provide adequate compensation for end-of-life care. The special circumstances of dying children—particularly the need for extended communication with children and parents, as well as health care team conferences—should be taken into account in setting reimbursement levels and in actually paying claims for these services when providers bill for them.

Information on palliative and end-of-life care is largely absent from materials developed for the public about cancer treatment. In addition, reliable information about survival from different types and stages of cancer is not routinely included with treatment information.

Recommendation 5: Organizations that provide information about cancer treatment (NCI, the American Cancer Society, and other patient-oriented organizations [e.g., disease-specific groups]; health insurers; and pharmaceutical companies) should revise their inventories of patient-oriented material, as appropriate, to provide comprehensive, accurate information about palliative care throughout the course of disease. Patients would also be helped by having reliable information on survival by type and stage of cancer easily accessible. Attention should be paid to cultural relevance and special populations (e.g., children).

Practice guidelines for palliative care and for other end-of-life issues are in comparatively early stages of development, and quality indicators are even more embryonic. Progress toward their further development and implementation requires continued encouragement by professional societies, funding bodies, and payers of care.

Recommendation 6: Best available practice guidelines should dictate the standard of care for both physical and psychosocial symptoms. Care systems, payers, and standard-setting and accreditation bodies should strongly encourage their expedited development, validation, and use. Professional societies, particularly the American Society of Clinical Oncology, the Oncology Nursing Society, and the Society for Social Work Oncology, should encourage their members to facilitate the development and testing of guidelines and their eventual implementation, and should provide leadership and training for nonspecialists, who provide most of the care for cancer patients.

Recommendation 7: The recommendations in the NCPB report Enhancing Data Systems to Improve the Quality of Cancer Care (see Appendix B) should be applied equally to palliative and end-of-life care as to other aspects of cancer treatment. These recommendations include

- *developing a core set of cancer care quality measures;*
- *increasing public and private support for cancer registries;*
- *supporting research and demonstration projects to identify new mechanisms to organize and finance the collection of data for cancer care quality studies;*
- *supporting the development of technologies, including computer-based patient record systems and intranet-based communication systems, to improve the availability, quality, and timeliness of clinical data relevant to assessing quality of cancer care;*
- *expanding support for training in health services research and other disciplines needed to measure quality of care;*
- *increasing support for health services research aimed toward improved quality of cancer care measures;*
- *developing models for linkage studies and the release of confidential data for research purposes that protect the confidentiality and privacy of health care information; and*
- *funding demonstration projects to assess the impact of quality monitoring programs within health care systems.*

Research on palliative care for cancer patients has had a low priority at NCI, and as a result, few researchers have been attracted to the field and very few relevant studies have been funded over the past decades. NCI should continue to collaborate on end-of-life research with the National Institute of Nursing Research (the lead NIH institute for this topic) but cannot discharge its major responsibilities in cancer research through that mechanism.

Recommendation 8: NCI should convene a State of the Science Meeting[1] on palliative care and symptom control. It should invite other National Institutes of Health, and government research agencies with shared interests should be invited to collaborate. The meeting should result in a high-profile strategic research agenda that can be pursued by NCI and its research partners over the short and long terms.

---

[1]In 1999, NCI initiated State of the Science Meetings focused on specific types of cancer "to bring together the Nation's leading multidisciplinary experts, to identify the important research questions for a given disease and help define the scientific research agenda that will assist us in addressing those questions."

Recommendation 9: NCI should establish the most appropriate institutional locus (or more than one) for palliative care, symptom control, and other end-of-life research, possibly within the Division of Cancer Treatment and Diagnosis.

Recommendation 10: NCI should review the membership of its advisory bodies to ensure representation of experts in cancer pain, symptom management, and palliative care.

References

Agency for Healthcare Research and Quality (AHRQ). 2001. *Management of Cancer Pain.* Summary, Evidence Report/Technology Assessment: Number 35. AHRQ Publication No. 01-E033, January 20001. Rockville, MD: Agency for Healthcare Research and Quality. http://www.ahrq.gov/clinic/canpainsum.htm.

Ahmedzai S. 1998. Palliation of respiratory symptoms. In Doyle D, Hanks GWC, MacDonald N (eds.): *Oxford Textbook of Palliative Medicine* (2nd edition). New York: Oxford University Press; pp. 583-616.

American Society of Clinical Oncology (ASCO). Cancer care during the last phase of life. *JCO* 1998;16(5):1986-1996.

Begg L. NCI Cancer Training Branch. Personal communication to Hellen Gelband, June 2000.

Cassel CK, Foley KM. 1999. *Principles for Care of Patients at the End of Life: An Emerging Consensus among the Specialties of Medicine.* New York: Milbank Memorial Fund, 32 pp.

Christ GH, Sormanti M. Advancing social work practice in end-of-life care. *Social Work in Health Care* 1999;30(2):81-99.

Christakis NA, Escarce JJ. Survival of Medicare patients after enrollment in hospice programs. *New England Journal of Medicine* 1996;338:172-178.

Colbert K. National Cancer Institute Budget Office. Personal communication to Hellen Gelband, August 2000.

Donnelly S, Walsh D. The symptoms of advanced cancer. *Semin Oncol* 1995;22:67-72.

Emanuel, EJ. National Cancer Institute. Unpublished data, 2000.

Emanuel EJ, Fairclough D, Clarridge BC, Blum D, Bruera E, Penley WC, Schnipper LE, Mayer RJ. Attitudes and practices of U.S. oncologists regarding euthanasia and physician-assisted suicide. *Ann Intern Med* 2000a Oct 3;133(7):527-532.

Emanuel EJ, Fairclough DL, Slutsman J, Emanuel LL. Understanding economic and other burdens of terminal illness: the experience of patients and their caregivers. *Ann Intern Med* 2000b Mar 21;132(6):451-459.

Ferrell B, Virani R, Grant M, et al. Beyond the Supreme Court decision: nursing perspectives on end-of-life care. *Oncology Nursing Forum* 2000;27(3):445-455.

Freeman HP, Payne R. Racial injustice in health care. *New England Journal of Medicine* 2000;342:1045-1047.

Hilden JM, Emanuel EJ, Fairclough DL, Link MP, Foley KM, Clarridge BC, Schnipper LE, Mayer RJ. Attitudes and practices among pediatric oncologists regarding end-of-life care: results of the 1998 American Society of Clinical Oncology survey. *JCO* 2001;19:205-212.

Hogan C, Lynn J, Gabel J, Lunney J, O'Mara A, Wilkinson A. 2000 *A statistical profile of decedents in the Medicare program.* Washington, D.C., Medicare Payment Advisory Commission.

Hudgings C. National Institute on Nursing Research, personal communication to Hellen Gelband, 2000.

Institute of Medicine (IOM). 1997. *Approaching Death: Improving Care at the End of Life,* Field MJ, Cassel CK, eds. Washington, D.C.: National Academy Press.

IOM. 1999. *Ensuring Quality Cancer Care,* Hewitt M, Simone JV, eds. Washington, D.C.: National Academy Press.

IOM. 2000. *Enhancing Data Systems to Improve the Quality of Cancer Care,* Hewitt M, Simone JV, eds. Washington, D.C.: National Academy Press.

Joint Commission on Accreditation of Healthcare Organizations. Background on the Development of the Joint Commission Standards on Pain Management, July 31, 2000. JCAHO Web site, http://www.jcaho.org/trkhco_frm.html.

Lagnado L. Rules are rules: hospice's patients beat the odds, so Medicare decides to crack down—terminally ill who don't die within a 6-month period risk losing coverage—Al Ouimet's 9-year survival. *Wall Street Journal* June 5, 2000.

Medicare Payment Advisory Commission (MedPAC). 1999. *Report to the Congress: Selected Medicare Issues.* Washington, D.C.: MedPAC.

MedPAC. 2000. *Medicare Beneficiaries' Costs and Use of Care in the Last Year of Life.* Washington, D.C.: MedPAC.

Morrison RS, Wallenstein S, Natale DK, et al. "We don't carry that"—failure of pharmacies in predominantly nonwhite neighborhoods to stock opioid analgesics. *New England Journal of Medicine* 2000; 342:1023-1026.

NHPCO (National Hospice and Palliative Care Organization). Facts and figures on hospice care in America. NHPCO Web site, January 10, 2001. www.nhpco.org.

Pfeifer MP, et al. The discussion of end-of-life medical care by primary care patients and physicians: a multicenter study using structured qualitative interviews. *Journal of General Internal Medicine;* 1994;9(2):82-88.

Phillips RS, Hamel MB, Covinsky KE, Lynn J. Findings from SUPPORT and HELP: an introduction. *Journal of the American Geriatrics Society* 2000;48:S1-S5.

President's Cancer Panel. 1998. *Cancer Care Issues in the United States: Quality of Care, Quality of Life.* NCI Web site, http://deainfo.nci.nih.gov/ADVISORY/pcp/pcp97-98rpt/pcp97-98rpt.htm#letter.

Schroeder SA. The legacy of SUPPORT. *Annals of Internal Medicine* 1999;131(10):780-782.

Singer PA, Martin DK, Kelner M. Quality end of life care—patients' perspectives. *JAMA* 1999;281:163-168.

SUPPORT Principal Investigators. A controlled trial to improve care for seriously ill hospitalized patients. *JAMA* 1995;274(20):1591-1598.

World Health Organization. 1990. *Cancer Pain Relief and Palliative Care.* World Health Organization Technical Report Series 804. Geneva.

APPENDIX
A

TABLE A-1 NCI Funding for Palliative Care Research: Specific Projects Fiscal Year 1999

Total Project $	Percent[a]	$ Relevant to Palliative Care	Project Title[b]
603,532	100	603,532	Inhibition of Postoperative Gynecological Adhesions
364,549	100	364,549	Intelligent Knowledge Base for Cancer Pain Treatment
367,610	100	367,610	Diana2 Computer-Based Teaching of Elder Care
153,918	100	153,918	Palliative Training for Caregivers of Cancer Patients
133,702	100	133,702	Patterns Care for Cancer Patients at End of Life
103,382	100	103,382	Home Based Moderate Exercise for Breast Cancer Patients
117,792	100	117,792	Stress of Cancer Caregiving—Analysis and Intervention
602,537	100	602,537	Family Home Care for Cancer—A Community Based Model
70,464	100	70,464	Clinical Management of Cancer Pain in US Nursing Homes
500,685	100	500,685	Pain Measurement in Bone Marrow Transplantation
162,671	100	162,671	Method for the Analysis of Pain Clinical Trials
413,030	100	413,030	Laboratory Studies of Pain Control Methods
292,011	100	292,011	Cost Effectiveness of Lung Cancer Chemotherapy
360,637	100	360,637	Comparison of Psychosocial Intervention in Breast Cancer
498,233	100	498,233	Self Care Intervention to Control Cancer Pain
540,262	100	540,262	Breast Cancer—Preparing for Survivorship
175,615	100	175,615	Recycling of Urea Nitrogen in Cancer Cachexia
203,436	100	203,436	Adjustment to Breast Cancer
248,889	100	248,889	Clinical Investigations in Hodgkin's Disease
588,097	100	588,097	Cancer Pain and Its Management
1,205,625	100	1,205,625	Maximizing the Therapeutic Index of Childhood ALL
1,778,647	100	1,778,647	CCSP in Head and Neck Cancer Rehabilitation
8,747	100	8,747	Feasibility of Physioacoustic Therapy in Cancer Care
405,116	100	405,116	Pain and the Defense Response
79,000	100	79,000	Home Care Training for Younger Breast Cancer Patients

TABLE A-1 Continued

Total Project $	Percent[a]	$ Relevant to Palliative Care	Project Title[b]
358,290	100	358,290	A Simulator to Teach Therapeutic Communication Skills
412,812	100	412,812	Facilitating Positive Adaptation to Breast Cancer
416,067	100	416,067	Enhancing Recovery from Blood and Marrow Transplantation
451,385	100	451,385	Computerized Pain Report and Nursing Pain Consult Protocol
350,015	100	350,015	Item Banking and Cat for Quality of Life Outcomes
50,000	100	50,000	Menopausal Symptom Relief for Women with Breast Cancer
100,000	100	100,000	Exercise and Quality of Life in Women with Breast Cancer
99,975	100	99,975	Self Advocacy and Empowerment for Cancer Patients
100,000	100	100,000	Apoptosis Inhibitor for Alopecia Due to Cancer Therapy
99,805	100	99,805	Skin Patches for AIDS Patients
12,405	100	12,405	CCG Nursing Workshop—Challenges in CCG Nursing
74,918	100	74,918	Stress Reduction for Women with Breast Cancer
347,423	100	347,423	Gender Differences in Opioid Analgesia and Side Effects
363,294	100	363,294	Exercise—An Intervention for Fatigue in Cancer Patients
280,410	100	280,410	Cognitive Behavioral Aspects of Cancer Related Fatigue
404,999	100	404,999	Computerized Symptom Report Consult for Cancer Patients
328,624	100	328,624	Endothelin 1 Induced Pain and Metastatic Prostate Cancer
270,936	100	270,936	A Caregiver Intervention to Improve Hospice Outcomes
1,999,999	100	1,999,999	Center for Psycho-oncology Research
249,986	30	74,996	Longitudinal Quality of Life After Marrow Transplant
1,645,030	30	493,509	Epithelial Ovarian Cancer Program Project
2,441,974	30	732,592	Fluorescence Spectroscopy for Cervical Neoplasia
10,000	25	2,500	HIV, Leukemia, and Opportunistic Cancers
584,213	20	116,843	New Approaches to Brain Tumor Therapy CNS Consortium

continued on next page

TABLE A-1 Continued

Total Project $	Percent[a]	$ Relevant to Palliative Care	Project Title[b]
98,456	20	19,691	New Approaches to Brain Tumor Therapy CNS Consortium
290,809	20	58,162	Synthetic Studies on Tumor Promoters and Inhibitors
14,883	20	2,977	Technical Requirements for Image Guided Spine Procedures
1,578,050	15	236,708	National Black Leadership Initiative on Cancer
250,641	15	37,596	Quality of Life of Gynecologic Cancer Survivors
284,633	15	42,695	Prophylactic Mastectomy in Hereditary Breast Cancer
270,273	5	13,514	Depression, HPA Function and Smoking Abstinence in Women
TOTAL		**$18,331,326**	

NOTE: ALL = acute lymphocytic leukemia; CCG = Cancer Center Grant; CCSP = Cancer Control Science Program; CNS = central nervous system; HPA hypothalamic-pituitary-adrenal.

[a]NCI estimate of percent of total relevant to palliative care
[b]Grant numbers, principal investigators, and specific institutions have not been listed in this table.

SOURCE: Colbert, 2000.

TABLE A-2 NCI Funding for Palliative Care Research: Institutional Grants Fiscal Year 1999

Total Project $	Percent[a]	$ Relevant to Palliative Care	Project Title[b]
1,427,579	21.20	302,647	Great Lakes Regional Center for AIDS Research
1,682,639	21.20	356,719	Robert H Lurie Cancer Center
1,451,421	18.02	261,546	Cancer Center and Research Institute
554,090	10.63	58,900	University of Texas MD Anderson CCOP Research Base
781,064	10.37	80,996	Cancer Center Support Grant (CCSG)
2,018,050	10.00	201,805	SPORE in Breast Cancer
2,449,134	10.00	244,913	Bay Area Breast Cancer Translational Research Program
947,107	10.00	94,711	Cooperative Core Lab and Clinical Nutrition Research Unit
2,671,424	10.00	267,142	SPORE in Breast Cancer
409,734	8.23	33,721	Comprehensive Cancer Center—Wake Forest University Research Base Grant
1,182,855	6.11	72,272	ECOG CCOP Research Base
271,255	6.07	16,465	Scottsdale Community Clinical Oncology Program
209,774	6.07	12,733	San Juan Minority-Based Community Oncology Program
212,744	6.07	12,914	Cedar Rapids Oncology Project
199,707	6.07	12,122	Geisinger Clinical Oncology Program
262,463	6.07	15,932	Illinois Oncology Research Association CCOP
252,539	6.06	15,304	CCOP
218,728	6.06	13,255	Oklahoma CCOP
881,850	6.06	53,440	Metro Minnesota CCOP
359,450	6.06	21,783	Kalamazoo CCOP
481,448	6.06	29,176	Northern New Jersey Community Oncology Program
108,209	6.05	6,547	University of Michigan CCOP Research Base
455,553	6.05	27,561	CCOP—Colorado Cancer Research Program
269,121	6.05	16,282	Mainline Health CCOP
350,001	6.05	21,175	Toledo CCOP
424,715	6.05	25,695	Marshfield CCOP
483,525	6.05	29,253	Duluth CCOP
563,042	6.05	34,064	Carle Cancer Center CCOP
397,585	6.05	24,054	Meritcare Hospital CCOP
402,567	6.05	24,355	Sioux Community Cancer Consortium
359,785	6.04	21,731	Missouri Valley Cancer Consortium CCOP
399,670	6.04	24,140	Ann Arbor Regional CCOP
393,221	6.04	23,751	Ochsner CCOP
335,086	6.04	20,239	Iowa Oncology Research Association

continued on next page

TABLE A-2 Continued

Total Project $	Percent[a]	$ Relevant to Palliative Care	Project Title[b]
505,639	6.00	30,338	Clinical Oncology Program
350,433	6.00	21,026	Kansas City CCOP
273,234	6.00	16,394	University of Illinois Minority Based CCOP
445,098	6.00	26,706	Scott and White CCOP
434,322	6.00	26,059	Greenville, South Carolina CCOP
150,185	6.00	9,011	Gynecologic Oncology Group
296,456	6.00	17,787	Montana Cancer Consortium
185,244	6.00	11,115	Santa Rosa Memorial Hospital Regional CCOP
361,602	6.00	21,696	Hawaii Minority Based CCOP
301,593	6.00	18,096	South Texas Pediatric Minority Based CCOP
184,797	6.00	11,088	Minority Based Clinical Oncology Program
1,035,721	6.00	62,143	Southeast Cancer Control Consortium Inc.
500,180	6.00	30,011	Central Illinois CCOP
451,849	6.00	27,111	Mount Sinai CCOP
304,404	6.00	18,264	Tumor Institute CCOP
847,078	6.00	50,825	CCOP Research Base
165,969	6.00	9,958	CCSG Research Base for CCOP
501,148	6.00	30,069	Pediatric Oncology Group as a CCOP Research Base
510,286	6.00	30,617	Community Clinical Oncology Program
460,201	6.00	27,612	Southern Nevada Cancer Research Foundation CCOP
550,206	6.00	33,012	Northwest CCOP
761,255	6.00	45,675	North Shore CCOP
293,899	6.00	17,634	Greater Phoenix CCOP
462,893	6.00	27,774	Columbus CCOP
286,396	6.00	17,184	CCOP
266,547	6.00	15,993	Florida Pediatric CCOP
551,590	6.00	33,095	Upstate Carolina CCOP
3,877,581	6.00	232,655	CCOP—Biostatistical Center
405,949	6.00	24,357	Louisiana State University Medical Center Minority-Based CCOP
368,614	6.00	22,117	Virginia Commonwealth University Minority-Based CCOP
1,134,032	6.00	68,042	Cancer and Leukemia Group B CCOP Research Base
11,242,692	6.00	674,562	Southwest Oncology Group—CCOP Research Base
519,100	6.00	31,146	CCOP Research Base
1,568,634	6.00	94,118	CCOP
9,772,324	6.00	586,339	CCOP
240,240	6.00	14,414	Baptist Cancer Institute CCOP
406,637	6.00	24,398	Ozarks Regional CCOP
481,158	6.00	28,869	Atlanta Regional CCOP

TABLE A-2 Continued

Total Project $	Percent[a]	$ Relevant to Palliative Care	Project Title[b]
553,267	6.00	33,196	Christiana Care CCOP
425,939	6.00	25,556	Syracuse Hematology-Oncology CCOP
509,387	6.00	30,563	Columbia River Oncology Program
260,360	6.00	15,622	St Louis/Cape Girardeau CCOP
187,892	6.00	11,274	Green Mountain Oncology Group
400,043	6.00	24,003	Dayton Clinical Oncology Program
3,660,649	5.71	209,023	CCSG
6,026,463	4.63	279,025	Cancer Center Support (Core) Grant
6,756,815	3.34	225,678	Cancer Center Support
3,092,697	3.32	102,678	Cancer Center Core Support Grant
1,256,873	2.84	35,695	Cancer Center Support Grant
854,004	2.23	19,044	Cancer Center of Wake Forest University
5,818,218	1.37	79,710	CCSG
3,194,572	0.60	19,167	Cancer Center
2,056,974	0.44	9,051	CCSG
2,551,080	0.43	10,970	CCSG
2,220,205	0.41	9,103	Yale Comprehensive Cancer Center
4,876,435	0.30	14,629	Regional Oncology Research Center
3,510,542	0.21	7,372	CCSG
202,113	0.11	222	Genetic Markers for Therapy of Colon Cancer
2,640,213	0.11	2,904	ECOG Statistical Center—Data Management Office
2,329,568	0.11	2,563	ECOG Statistical Office
6,944,062	0.11	7,638	ECOG Operations Office
154,596	0.11	170	ECOG Institution Grant
181,018	0.11	199	ECOG
366,391	0.11	403	ECOG
281,735	0.11	310	ECOG
234,810	0.11	258	ECOG
446,441	0.11	491	ECOG
547,877	0.11	603	ECOG —Wisconsin Studies
393,987	0.11	433	ECOG Clinical Trials
286,855	0.11	316	ECOG
391,656	0.11	431	ECOG
170,319	0.11	187	ECOG
335,704	0.11	369	ECOG Studies
206,311	0.11	227	ECOG
426,499	0.11	469	ECOG
345,144	0.11	380	ECOG
742,780	0.11	817	ECOG Chair's Office
146,456	0.11	161	ECOG
3,001,469	0.05	1,501	University of Michigan Cancer Center

continued on next page

TABLE A-2 Continued

Total Project $	Percent[a]	$ Relevant to Palliative Care	Project Title[b]
2,865,494	0.02	573	American College of Surgeons Oncology Trials Group
824,877	0.02	165	Quality Assurance Review Center (QARC)
401,529	0.02	80	EORTC Data Center
735,000	0.02	147	Radiological Physics Center
2,803,329	0.02	561	CCSG
TOTAL		**6,148,591**	

NOTE: CCOP = Community Clinical Oncology Program; CCSG = Cancer Center Support Grant; ECOG = Eastern Cooperative Oncology Group; EORTC = European Organization for Research and Treatment of Cancer; SPORE = Specialized Program of Research Excellence.

[a]NCI estimate of percent of total relevant to palliative care

[b]Grant numbers, principal investigators, and specific institutions have not been listed in this table.

SOURCE: Colbert, 2000.

B
Recommendations from *Enhancing Data Systems to Improve the Quality of Cancer Care* (IOM, 2000)

1. Enhance Key Elements of the Data System Infrastructure

Recommendation 1: Develop a core set of cancer care quality measures.

The Secretary of the Department of Health and Human Services (DHHS) should designate a committee made up of representatives of public institutions (e.g., the DHHS Quality of Cancer Care Committee, state cancer registries, academic institutions) and private groups (e.g., consumer organizations, professional associations, purchasers, health insurers and plans) to: 1) identify a single core set of quality measures that span the full spectrum of an individual's care and are based on the best available evidence; 2) advise other national groups (e.g., National Committee for Quality Assurance, Joint Commission for the Accreditation of Healthcare Organizations, Quality Forum) to adopt the recommended core set of measures; and 3) monitor the progress of ongoing efforts to improve standard reporting of cancer stage and comorbidity.

a) Research sponsors (e.g., Agency for Healthcare Research and Quality [AHRQ], National Cancer Institute [NCI], Health Care Financing Administration [HCFA], Department of Veterans Affairs [VA]) should invest in studies to identify evidence-based quality indicators across the continuum of cancer care.

b) Ongoing efforts to standardize reporting of cancer stage and comorbidity should receive a high priority and be fully supported.

c) Efforts to identify quality of cancer care measures should be coordinated with ongoing national efforts regarding quality of care.

Recommendation 2: Congress should increase support to the Centers for Disease Control and Prevention (CDC) for the National Program of Cancer Registries (NPCR) to improve the capacity of states to achieve complete coverage and timely reporting of incident cancer cases. NPCR's primary purpose is cancer surveillance, but NPCR, together with the Surveillance, Epidemiology, and End Results (SEER) Program, has great potential to facilitate national, population-based assessments of the quality of cancer care through linkage studies and by serving as a sample frame for special studies.

Recommendation 3: Private cancer-related organizations should join the American Cancer Society and the American College of Surgeons to provide financial support for the National Cancer Data Base. Expanded support would facilitate efforts underway to report quality benchmarks and performance data to institutions providing cancer care.

Recommendation 4: Federal research agencies (e.g., NCI, CDC, AHRQ, HCFA) should support research and demonstration projects to identify new mechanisms to organize and finance the collection of data for cancer care quality studies. Current data systems tend to be hospital based, while cancer care is shifting to outpatient settings. New models are needed to capture entire episodes of care, irrespective of the setting of care.

Recommendation 5: Federal research agencies (e.g., National Institutes of Health [NIH], Food and Drug Administration [FDA], CDC, and VA) should support public-private partnerships to develop technologies, including computer-based patient record systems and intranet-based communication systems, that will improve the availability, quality, and timeliness of clinical data relevant to assessing quality of cancer care.

Recommendation 6: Federal research agencies (e.g., NCI, AHRQ, VA) should expand support for training in health services research and training of professionals with expertise in the measurement of quality of care and the implementation and evaluation of interventions designed to improve the quality of care.

2. Expand Support for Analyses of Quality of Cancer Care
Using Existing Data Systems

Recommendation 7: Federal research agencies (e.g., NCI, AHRQ, VA) should expand support for health services research, especially studies based on the linkage of cancer registry to administrative data and special studies of cases sampled from cancer registries. Resources should also be made available through NPCR and SEER to provide technical assistance to states to help them expand the capability of using cancer registry data for quality improvement initiatives. NPCR should also be supported in its efforts to consolidate state data and link them to national data files.

Recommendation 8: Federal research agencies (e.g., NCI, AHRQ, HCFA) should develop models for the conduct of linkage studies and the release of confidential data for research purposes that protect the confidentiality and privacy of healthcare information.

3. Monitor the Effectiveness of Data Systems to Promote Quality
Improvement Within Health Systems.

Recommendation 9: Federal research agencies (e.g., NCI, AHRQ, HCFA, VA) should fund demonstration projects to assess the application of quality monitoring programs within healthcare systems and the impact of data-driven changes in the delivery of services on the quality of health care. Findings from the demonstrations should be disseminated widely to consumers, payers, purchasers, and cancer care providers.

Acronyms and Abbreviations

ACS	American Cancer Society
AHRQ	Agency for Healthcare Research and Quality
ASCO	American Society of Clinical Oncology
CIS	Cancer Information Service
DCTD	Division of Cancer Treatment and Diagnosis
HCFA	Health Care Financing Administration
HELP	Hospitalized Elderly Longitudinal Project
HRSA	Health Resources and Services Administration
IOM	Institute of Medicine
JCAHO	Joint Commission on Accreditation of Healthcare Organizations
MDS	Minimum Data Set
MedPAC	Medicare Payment Advisory Commission
NCCN	National Comprehensive Cancer Network
NCI	National Cancer Institute
NCPB	National Cancer Policy Board
NIAID	National Institute of Allergy and Infectious Diseases

NIH   National Institutes of Health
NINR   National Institute of Nursing Research
NMFBS   National Mortality Followback Survey

PCP   President's Cancer Panel
PDIA   Project on Death in America
PDQ   Physician Data Query

RWJF   Robert Wood Johnson Foundation

SEER   Surveillance, Epidemiology, and End Results Program
SUPPORT   Study to Understand Prognoses and Preferences for
               Outcomes and Risks of Treatment

VA   Department of Veterans Affairs

WHO   World Health Organization